W9-AUY-331

LIMBO

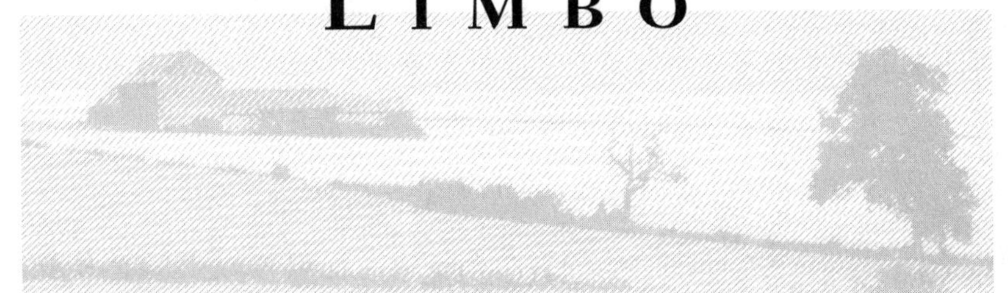

Also by A. Manette Ansay

Vinegar Hill

Read This and Tell Me What It Says

Sister

River Angel

Midnight Champagne

LIMBO

A MEMOIR

A. Manette Ansay

wm

WILLIAM MORROW 75 YEARS OF PUBLISHING

An Imprint of HarperCollins*Publishers*

FIRST EDITION

Designed by Jo Anne Metsch

Printed on acid-free paper

Library of Congress Cataloging-in-Publication Data has been applied for.

ISBN 0-688-17286-5

01 02 03 04 05 QW 10 9 8 7 6 5 4 3 2 1

This book is dedicated to the first novel
I loved: *The Chosen* by Chaim Potok

Contents

Acknowledgments

I would like to thank the MacDowell Colony, where a chunk of this book was written. Heartfelt thanks to Oprah Winfrey and her book club for what has amounted to an incredible arts grant at a time when I needed it most.

Family members appear in *Limbo* under their own names, because they have lived this with me, and I wanted them beside me on the page. However, the names of acquaintances, teachers, and people with whom I've lost touch have been changed.

This is, to the best of my ability, a book of nonfiction. However, this does not mean that someone else might not remember or interpret things differently. Every experience consists of many stories and many points of view. This one happens to be mine.

LIMBO

Prologue: 1975

In fifth grade, they divided us for the afternoon. The boys were sent to the gym to play kickball, while we girls crowded into the windowless room next door. The school nurse was there, and so was the guidance counselor, along with a lady we had never seen before. She wore makeup and a tall blond wig, and she was busy setting up a film projector.

The kickballs *thunk-thunked* like distant drums.

"This is going to be gross," my best friend, Tabitha, said.

In fourth grade, she'd told me what Keri Hommerding had told her: that to make a baby, a man stuck his thing up inside you, *there*. "That's not true," I insisted, but just to make sure, I checked with my mother. Instead of denying it, as I fully expected her to do, she'd sighed and removed the pins from her mouth—she'd been sewing a Halloween costume for my brother—and said that there were beautiful explanations of conception and then there were ugly ones, and that Keri Hommerding's was one of the ugly ones. She said that before I was born, she and my father both had gone to church and prayed very hard that God would send them a baby, and because they were very much in love with each other, God had sent them my brother and me.

It was so unlike my mother to lie that both of us blushed until my mother said, "OK?" and put the pins back in her mouth. I crept out of the room, feeling sick to my stomach, for I knew that the truth had to exist in some terrible in-between place. That night, just as I was falling asleep, it came to me like an incubus. It sat on my chest and sucked my breath and there was absolutely nothing I could do. Sex was what Father Stone did to people in the confessional. Hadn't I seen all the mothers and fathers lining up to see him, week after week? Hadn't I watched them step, one by one, behind the red velvet curtain? Hadn't I always wondered what *really* went on in there?

"Are you sure you want a baby?" Father Stone would say, pulling up his long, loose frock under which—all the kids would have bet their lives on this—he wore absolutely nothing at all. "Will you be good parents?"

I'd tried to put the whole business out of my head, but now that my First Confession was drawing near, it was often on my mind. Once, I'd asked my mother if I might delay my First Confession until I was older, but she'd replied that I was mature for my age. In her opinion, I was ready.

"Ladies," said the lady in the tall, blond wig. Her voice was calm, respectful. A frenzy of kickballs battered the wall; she paused until the sound subsided. "Your bodies are going to start changing soon. Your hips will widen. You'll develop breasts. You'll notice hair growing in places you never had hair before. Some of you may already have noticed some or all of these changes."

"Barf," I whispered to Tabitha.

"I told you," Tabitha said.

But the film the blond lady showed wasn't gross at all. It was a cartoon, and it was very funny, with this wild-eyed crazy sperm darting around after an egg who, looking bored, batted her very long eyelashes. And after the film, each of us got a paper bag of gifts: Kotex of various sizes, a pink, pocket-size calendar, and a slender, matching pen. *Very Personally Yours* was written in gold script across the front of each calendar. The lady explained how to mark the calendars on the first day of our periods, how to calculate when ovulation—the release of an egg—would occur. During ovulation, we could become pregnant if we engaged in sexual intercourse. Did we all know what sexual intercourse was?

Nobody breathed. I imagined Father Stone's red-knuckled hands tugging his robe up over his knees.

"Sexual intercourse occurred when a husband put his penis inside his wife's vagina and moved it rapidly back and forth," the lady said. The friction was enjoyable to both. Sperm came out of the husband's penis and fertilized the wife's egg.

Next door, the boys cheered. Somebody had scored.

"Do you have to be married?" Martha Sheinke asked.

"Yes," the lady said.

All around me, girls were murmuring squeamishly, but I thought I might faint with relief. The lady's voice was so calm, so matter-of-fact, that I knew she was telling the truth. My First Confession would be fine now, it wouldn't be any big deal. I wouldn't have to have sexual intercourse until I got married, and Father Stone would have nothing to do with it.

Did anyone have any questions?

Adrenaline fired through my veins. My hand shot joyfully into the air before I realized it had done so.

"Yes?"

I leaped to my feet. I was grinning, an ear-to-ear foolish grin. All the other girls were looking at me. I didn't know what to say.

"Yes?" the lady said again.

"Can you sleep on your stomach if you're pregnant?" I blurted.

Everybody laughed and I laughed, too, only then I kept on laughing. I couldn't stop. I couldn't sit down. Tears leaked from the corners of my eyes. The other girls looked at me uneasily.

"Can you sleep on your stomach if you're pregnant?" the lady repeated soothingly, as if she understood. "Now that's a good one. I don't know if I can answer that because I've never been pregnant. Do either of you have children?" she asked the school nurse and the guidance counselor. But neither of them did.

"It is probably safe to use common sense," the lady said, "and assume that the answer is no."

Part One

One

I have moved eleven times in the sixteen years since leaving *home,* a word that to me will always mean southeastern Wisconsin, and the little town where I was raised, and my grandmother's one-hundred-acre farm seven miles to the north. At thirty-six, wading through the shallows of middle age, I have been permanently shaped—and am still held fast—by landscapes that exist in memory alone, though this makes them no less real when they come to me in dreams, when fragments are triggered by a random fact or phrase. Here is my body's lost exuberance. Here is my Catholic faith, that Gothic cathedral, that haunted house. Here are the straight highways, the crops and their seasons, the blue haze of Lake Michigan: wide-open space beneath a close sky.

It doesn't take much—a look, a phrase—and suddenly I'm a child once more, running hard and fast down a narrow dirt road that has since been developed into another antiseptic side street, the fallow fields surrounding it sold, subdivided, populated by three-bedroom ranch houses, each wrapped in vinyl the color of a hospital gown, each with its garage door shut, an expressionless face, like someone waiting for bad news. Yet there's no sense, as I run, that I'm re-creating something, repainting this landscape as if by numbers, filling in color and sound. I'm simply *here,* I'm *home,* and any return to the present will be informed by what I've seen.

How is it that, for this splendid moment, I'm *able* to run—something I haven't done since I was twenty—elbows pumping, heels striking the earth, carrying myself deeper into a place that is nowhere, nothing, lost, in a body whose unselfconscious sense of movement, whose entitlement to such movement, is lost as well? The part in my hair feels like a cut where the August sun strikes against it, the skin tingling pink. There's a sweet, cold ache in my chest, a lemonade taste in my mouth. I feel as if I could run forever, but, of course, I'm wrong. When the ball of my foot meets a stone, I suck in my breath and hop toward the ditch, where I collapse matter-of-factly to inspect the damage.

A coin of blood, bright as a posy. In its center, a pebble. A scrutinizing eye.

Automatically, I offer my thanks to God, my pain to the Poor Souls in Purgatory. The pebble is God's message, His communication, His way of making me pay attention; I study it the way I'd study a difficult problem at school. *Give thanks in all circumstances,* the Bible says. Perhaps, the pebble kept me from running ahead into the path of a rattlesnake sunning itself in the dust. Perhaps, the pebble has delayed me just long enough to prevent me from crossing Holden Street, where I live, as a speeding car hurtles through. In my world, in the deep, underwater sleep of belief, there is no such thing as an accident. Just because you can't find the reason doesn't mean it isn't there. God is simply testing you, testing the condition of your Faith.

I imagine my Faith like a diamond or ruby, a shining, precious stone. Something that must be protected. Something that can be shattered, stolen, lost. A person who loses their Faith, I know, becomes an *atheist.* The sound of the word gives me the feeling I get when, at slumber parties, my friends and I sneak outside. We walk through the darkness in our flimsy nightgowns, pretending there is somebody following just behind us, a man dressed in black and holding a knife. We can feel his hot breath on our shoulders. We can hear him licking his lips. We stare straight ahead, taking slow deliberate steps, for he's unable to touch any of us—

as long as we all stick together. As long as nobody looks back.

I stand up, brush off my shorts, eager to head back home. Already, the pebble is a story I can tell, a currency to be spent. I'll walk all the way to Holden Street on my heel, careful not to jar the pebble loose. There, I'll find my younger brother and make him watch me dig it out. If he's admiring, I'll let him keep it. If he feigns indifference, I'll tell him about tetanus, enact the grim onset of symptoms, suck my cheeks hollow as starvation sets in. When he's on the verge of telling our mother, tears bright in his eyes, I'll admit that I've had a tetanus shot.

Then, with slow relish, I'll describe the length of the needle, how the nurse shoved it in, to the bone.

"**The cradle rocks** above an abyss," Vladamir Nabokov writes, "and common sense tells us that our existence is but a brief crack of light between two eternities of darkness."

Memory, then, like the switch on the wall. The pull chain on the lamp.

My first memory is of memory itself—and the fear of its loss, that vast outer dark.

One night, as I lay floating in the still, dark pond between wakefulness and sleep, a stray thought breached the surface like a fish. *You will forget this.* I opened my eyes. To my right, tucked under the covers beside me, was an eyeless Raggedy Ann doll. To my left, on top of the covers, was a large plastic spark plug—a display model that my father, a traveling salesman, had coaxed from some farm dealership and presented to me. My father's gifts were unpredictable and strange: hotel ashtrays, pens with company slogans trailing down their sides, desiccated frogs and snakes he found along the highway, jaws pulled back in agonized smiles. These things populated the bedroom I shared with my two-year-old brother like the grasshoppers and pianos and clocks in a Dali painting, startling the eye from my mother's homemade curtains, the Infant of Prague night-light keeping watch on the bedside table, the child-size rocking chair. The spark plug was nearly three feet long; if you shook it, something mysterious rattled around inside. It was tied by a string to a wooden spool and, during the day, I dragged it clattering after me, the way other girls carried dolls.

You will forget this.

It was 1969. I was four years old, almost five. The thought swam back and forth in the darkness, gaining speed, and I could see it was an ugly thing, long as the moray eel in the *World Book Encyclopedia,* with rows of needle-sharp teeth. Fully awake now, I sat up, swung my legs off the edge of the bed. Could it be true? Across the room, my brother slept in the crib that had once been mine. It was the size of a generous icebox, the wood-slatted sides painted light green, and I could not imagine being small enough to sleep comfortably inside it. Yet my mother had pictures to prove that I had, slides I could hold up to the light. A solemn-eyed baby stared back at me. *You,* my mother explained. She said that Mike wouldn't remember being a baby, either. Nobody did.

At the time, we were renting a house in Michigan, forty miles from Detroit. Piggyback trucks rattled over the speed bump on the highway, twenty feet from our porch; railroad tracks divided the gray-faced neighborhood. At night, the slow-moving freight trains passed so close that I could feel the vibrations in my mattress, my chest. It was a sensation I loved. Would there be trains in Wisconsin? I'd wanted to know when my mother explained we would be moving there in May, returning to the area where she and my father had grown up, where their parents and brothers and sisters still lived. Already, she'd started boxing things up. During the day, I wandered from room to room, passing my hands through the empty spaces where, only weeks earlier, the pieces of my life had exhibited themselves, unquestionable as the prayers I said before and after each meal, incontrovertible as God.

Now, to test myself, I imagined everything back where it belonged. I went through the small dark rooms of my memory, moving myself like a game piece, forcing myself to articulate everything I saw, or heard, or smelled, or touched. How could I forget our kitchen with its chipped Formica counter, or the picnic table where we ate, painted pale blue—the Virgin's color—and built into the wall? Or my parents' bedroom with its neat twin beds, and the way I'd catch them holding hands across the open space between them? The morning light coming in through the "sheers"—pale, fancy curtains that I wasn't allowed to touch. The look and feel of my hands just as they were, the right one finally big enough to span a major fourth on the piano.

Everything was there for me, safe in its place. Even the darkness was familiar, bound to the sound of my brother's sleep, his tapioca smell.

Still, just to be sure, I re-created the previous day: rising, dressing, eating breakfast, walking to nursery school with my mother, home again for lunch and a nap, then late afternoon at the piano, and supper, and a bath, and bedtime. I recited, word for word, the books my mother had read to me; I listed the foods I'd eaten. But some parts of the day were less clear than others, and when I attempted to recapture an earlier day with the same intensity, I faltered. Suddenly, I thought of all the times I'd begged my mother to tell me what she'd been like at my age: the first word she'd learned to read, the first song she'd learned to play on the piano.

"I don't remember," she'd say. Or, "That was a long time ago."

The truth hit me then: I *would* forget. There was nothing I could do. Someday, I'd be a grown-up woman, and I'd forget all about the girl I was now. It would be as if she'd never existed. I extended my legs, pink in the night-light's glow, and they seemed otherworldly, unattached. Years later, reading *Slaughterhouse-Five,* I encountered Kurt Vonnegut's famous line: *"Listen: Billy Pilgrim has come unstuck in time,"* and I saw myself, again, on that night, in that room, and at last I had the words to describe exactly what I'd felt.

"I feel stupid," was what I told my mother then, and on the nights that followed, when she'd get up to find out why I'd turned on the light, why I wasn't sleeping.

"But you're *smart,*" she'd say, and we'd stare at each other, despairing, for I was unable to explain what I meant, and she couldn't imagine what was wrong. As soon as she'd leave, I'd sit up again, because without the light, I knew I'd fall asleep. And I didn't want to sleep. I had work to do. I was trying to save us all. By day, my mother was packing up the house; at night, I packed again, in secret. I memorized the layout of the house, the arrangement of the furniture, the furniture itself. In my mind's eye, I opened the kitchen cupboards, the bedroom closets, the vanity over the bathroom sink. I marched around the backyard, marking the location of trees, noting the imperfections of the swing set. I sat down at the piano and went over the simple songs I'd learned, and the long melody played with both hands in unison that I was endlessly composing. Then I recited events, beginning with the most recent day and working my way back in time as far as I could. After a week or so, this litany became like a prayer, a sequence of words I could rattle off without thinking, the syllables slurred, the intonations unvaried.

The trouble was this: with each passing day, new events had to be added. This made the litany grow longer and longer. At nursery school, I sat quietly, trying to limit the things I'd be obliged to remember that night. My mother took me to see Dr. Heitch, and I sat on a table covered in white paper, staring down at his bright green pants, which reminded me of Mr. Greenjeans on Captain Kangaroo. This detail, too, was duly noted, packaged in a coil of words, sealed and labeled for the future. Someday, the grown-up person I'd become might want this image back. She might, for whatever unforeseen reason, decide she needed these things I was storing away with an archivist's care. And if she did, they would be waiting for her, just like our plates and cups and photographs would be waiting for us when we got to Wisconsin, wrapped up in pieces of newspaper.

We moved in June, first to my maternal grandmother's farm for the summer, and then, at the end of August, to my paternal grandparents' house in the nearby town of Port Washington, where we lived while our house on Holden Street was being built. One evening after supper, my father took my brother and me to see the newly poured foundation. He pointed out where the walls would go, and the stairs leading up to the second story. The house would have wall-to-wall carpeting, a two-car garage, central heat. From now on, we'd even have our own bedrooms—what did we think of that?

"The Tiger needs his own cage," he said, dropping a hand on my brother's shoulder.

Within a few weeks, the house had floors. The skeleton of walls appeared and then, remarkably, walls themselves, with copper pipes and insulation and Sheetrock. There was a fireplace big enough to sit in. Ceiling fixtures. Toilets. We brought scraps of lumber back to my grandparents' house and carried them down to the basement where my grandmother never went. There we played for hours, designing houses, then knocking them down. Upstairs, my grandmother sat in her chair, strangling her rosary between her long, white fingers.

I no longer lay awake at night, trying to remember things, perhaps because there was nothing about my grandparents' house I particularly wanted to remember. Still, I clung to the old litany, chanted it as if it were a charm, a magical incantation as I fidgeted through the Lawrence Welk Show, as I sat through my grandparents' endless mealtime bickering, as I stared up into the bright orange clusters of berries that hung from the small, regularly spaced trees in front of my grandparents' house. The berries were poisonous, my mother explained. They were *decorative* berries, which meant they were there to look at, not to eat. At my other grandmother's farm, there had been mulberries, gooseberries, raspberries, blackberries. I'd eaten my fill of them and beyond, eaten until my lips were raw, sour-tasting against the sweet, and my other grandmother had laughed whenever I'd stuck out my brilliant red tongue.

One day, it occurred to me that each of my grandmothers had the *right kind* of berries. I tried to explain this to my mother, but without the word *symbol,* we wound up exchanging another round of despairing looks. Yet the thought left me wonderfully satisfied. It was delicious, like solving a puzzle, like having the last word.

In September, I started kindergarten. My father began to travel again, and in his absence, my grandparents left all the cooking and cleaning and laundry to my mother. She had just started a new job herself, teaching fifth grade at the same public school I attended, and her utter exhaustion made her seem unreal, a copy of a copy of herself. Whenever I could, I lingered near my classroom door, hoping to catch a glimpse of her walking past in the hall. "Are you my mother?" I'd ask. "Are you sure?" She'd laugh and kiss me, tickle my neck, thinking I was playing a game.

At noon, when my school day ended, I'd walk back to my grandparents' house with another little girl who lived on the same street. My brother always waited for me in the front bay window. He'd follow me around as I got out two plates, poured two glasses of milk, divided the sandwich my mother had left for us. My grandmother watched, clicking her tongue. She prepared and ate her own food. "Naughty girl," she'd tell me for no reason I could see, and a strange little smile fluttered about her lips. My grandfather was seldom home with us. He left every morning for the senior citizens' center, where he spent the day playing sheepshead and gin rummy. In his absence, my grandmother would say peculiar things. "I know all about you," she'd whisper, nodding with narrowed eyes, as if she were seeing someone else, someone she didn't like. Sometimes she cried for no reason. Sometimes she told my brother he was really her little boy.

One day, my brother wasn't waiting for me in the window. I found him in the spare room. He was under the blankets on the daybed, sucking his thumb, staring at nothing. I talked to him for a long time before he finally blinked, disbelieving, like a very old man awakened from a charmed and terrible sleep. My grandmother had told him that my mother was dead. It had never occurred to me that an adult, a grown-up person, might tell a lie. Suddenly, the world gained a whole new perspective. Sentences cast long shadows in which anything might hide. I listened with new ears, spoke with a fresh tongue. At school, if somebody asked what I'd had for breakfast, and I'd had eggs, I'd say, "Cereal." Why? Just because I could. Just to see if anything happened. Nothing ever did. How easily one word could be swapped for another. How effortlessly you could build a secret life, a second life, a kind of shelter.

At last our house was ready. We moved in, unpacked our belongings, settled into our new lives. My mind was occupied with school, and as I grew older, I became more interested in learning new things than remembering old ones. Gradually, I let go of the litany I'd loved, each detail linked so deliberately to the next, all those things I'd packed away in secret. Over time, they were shoved further and further to the back of my consciousness. I doubt I'd ever have found them if I hadn't, in my early twenties, fallen ill.

Two

This is the story that, for more than ten years, I could not tell, the single thing my father asked me not to write about.

On a clear, cold day in January 1955, my grandfather drove my father to a tuberculosis sanatorium in Plymouth, Wisconsin, where he would remain for the next twenty months. My father was nineteen. He had a ninth-grade education. He carried a bundle containing his pajamas, a bathrobe, bed linens, a single towel. No personal items. No magazines or books, for even if there had been such things in my grandparents' house, my father would not have thought to read them. He followed the nurse, Miss Monica, to the bed that had been prepared for him, the last bed at the end of a long row of beds, some of which were curtained, some of which were occupied by sallow-faced women. A few of these women slept. Others followed him with their eyes. One of them winked.

"None of that," Miss Monica said.

She explained that this, the ground floor, was the women's ward. The men's ward spanned the three upper floors, which were overcrowded and noisy. The men assigned to the highest floor, according to Miss Monica, were *wild—so* wild, in fact, that two had only recently crawled out the windows, scaled the walls like monkeys, and vanished into the trees. Considering my father's youth, Miss Monica thought it would be best if he claimed a bed in the women's ward. Things would be quieter here. She reminded him how important it was that he lie flat, keep still. Medication would help him sleep. A TV rotated between the floors; each floor got it, in its turn, for one week.

After she'd gone, my father pulled the curtain around his bed. He undressed and lay down. After a while, he reached out and tugged the curtain back. The woman who had winked at him winked again. My father closed his eyes. He would celebrate his next two birthdays in this room, in this bed.

Tuberculosis was not uncommon in rural Wisconsin. No

doubt my father contracted it through a carrier who had gotten it from his cattle, as did so many of the farmers in those days. The TB settled in their lungs, or in their joints, or in their spines. Absolute bed rest, along with antibiotics and isolation, was the standard treatment of the day. Under these conditions, the body fought the disease by gradually containing it within a calcified node. At that point, the growth could be surgically removed—in my father's case, more than a year after he'd first been admitted to the san.

The san. My father describes the day he was admitted in the careful, paint-by-numbers tones of a man not used to revealing personal things. It is his gift to me. "A clear day," he says. "Clear and cold. January twenty-first, 1955."

He is standing in the doorway of my bedroom, halfway in, halfway out. It's early evening, just after supper, and I'm already back in bed, where I've spent most of the day. Lumps the size of frozen peas have buckled my shins, and even the short trek from the dining room has left every muscle below my knees burning. Crutches help support my weight, but I can't use them for long because my wrists and forearms are also inflamed. I lie rigid under ice packs, the bedside lamp turned out.

It is 1987. I am twenty-two years old. Walking, gripping a cup, standing up long enough to take a shower—simple things like these are agony, and no one can explain why. Three years earlier, I'd been forced to drop out of the

Peabody Conservatory of Music, where I was a piano performance major, unable to control the inflammation in my arms and hands. After casting about for another career, I wound up at the University of Maine—the result of a series of drifting, short-term jobs—and there I took courses in genetics, evolution, anthropology, trying to reinvent myself, to imagine a life without music at its core. It was easy, at first, to ignore the fact that my health continued to deteriorate. Then I began to limp. I dropped things. I fell down. Finally, I took a medical leave, expecting to be back in a month, maybe two.

By now, fifteen months have passed.

Twice, I've attempted to return to school, to get to my classes on crutches; twice I've been forced to pack up and go home. On a good day, I can crutch the length of the house; on a bad day, I stay in bed, avoiding liquids so I won't have to haul myself to the bathroom, waiting for my mother to come home from work, which she does twice a day, to see if I need anything. She touches my hair, asks me questions, forces me to interact with the human world. On weekends, she helps me out to the car, heaves the folding wheelchair we've leased from a drugstore into the trunk, and takes me to Cedar Grove for an ice cream, to Brown Deer for a movie. She suggests foreign language tapes, educational videos, correspondence classes. She buys me a tape recorder and cassettes so I can record the college assignments my hands cannot write, the papers I'm supposed to be turning in by mail.

Nights after supper, when my mother comes into my room, she throws on all the lights, sets up the Scrabble board. But my father stands helpless in the doorway. He does not turn on the light. Halfway in and halfway out, he tells his story, this story, the one he never talked about when, as a child, I asked questions. He describes the same details again and again: the squirrels that came to the window. The slow rotation of the TV. The man upstairs who wept each night until the others shouted him into silence.

My father's body forms the shape of a star against the bright backdrop of the hall. In the months since my illness began, our relationship has changed. Before, he was simply *Dad,* a stock character, like somebody on TV: the breadwinner, the tie-breaker, the one who threatened to put his foot down. You applied to him for money, or if you needed to borrow the car. Facts rattled in his pockets like change. One of those facts, of course, was *love,* but this was a coin that never got spent, one that stayed deep in the safety of his pocket, for the world of emotion was my mother's terrain. But now all of that has been swept away. My father holds nothing back. He describes the slow passage of days, his exhaustion, his bewilderment. If I cry, he doesn't leave the room but stays, the way my mother stays: waiting, weathering, solid ground.

And when he tells me that someday what is happening to me will feel like a dream, like it happened to somebody else, I do not get angry the way that I do when other people, trying to cheer me, say the same thing. I don't ask, *How can you pretend to know how I will feel?* I don't say, *This time is all lost for good, and even if I get better someday, I will never get this part of my life back, don't you see?* I don't ask, *And what if I don't get better, what if things just go on and on the way they are?* which is all I think about during the long hours when he and my mother are both at work and my friends no longer call, when relatives and neighbors and people from our church go about their own lives, as they should, as they must, though they remember me—they are quick to assure my mother after Mass—in their prayers.

My maternal grandmother lights candles for me, buys Masses to be said in Rome on my behalf. An aunt wants to send me to Boston, to a priest who heals by laying-on of hands. Everybody says they are praying for me. Everybody tells me that God has His reasons, that everything is part of His plan. But I no longer believe in God that way, as someone who cares about any one person's problems, an almighty mechanic who charges stiff fees to repair what was in His all-knowing plan to break.

Alone in my room. Time doesn't pass. It bleeds, blurs, washes me along. Sometimes, I strap braces on my wrists and poke at the typewriter my mother has placed on a card table next to my bed. She encourages me to write poetry, to identify the birds that visit the window feeder, to read the dog-eared books she brings from our limited public library. She is still looking for that silver lining. She believes—fiercely, inconsolably—that we have every reason to be optimistic, that the cup is actually half full. But I can't raise my feet or point my toes. I can't grip a pen. I have blood in my stool. I'm in constant pain, and though I can't imagine how this can be, everything seems to be getting worse.

There have been, of course, many theories over the course of the past fifteen months. There have been, along with each of these theories, their attendant diagnostic procedures. Another clinic. Another doctor. Another bill with its neat, itemized columns.

I am told I have lupus. I have a viral infection. I have heavy metal poisoning, environmental illness, food allergies. I am psychosomatically ill. I have Hodgkin's disease. I am experiencing aftereffects from a concussion I had when I was twelve. I have systematic tendinitis, fibromyalgia. I have a chronic pain syndrome, a rheumatoid disorder, sympathetic reflex dystrophy, peripheral neuropathy, a reaction that harks back to an overprescription of penicillin during my teens. I *might* have MS, but it's too soon to say, we'll just have to wait and see.

I have tests and more tests: bone scans, nerve conduction studies, MRI's, dozens of X rays. I have neurological exams in which I close my eyes, touch my index finger to my nose, attempt to stand on one foot. I have psychiatric exams in which I'm asked if I hear voices. I have rheumatoid exams in which the same blood tests are repeated again and again. I have ultrasound treatments, paraffin dips, TENS, biofeedback, injections of B vitamins. I have endless physical therapy, which inevitably makes things worse, for any repetitive activity involving my arms or legs causes still more inflammation. At a university "teaching" hospital, I have an exquisitely painful lumbar block—"to restart your neurological system," I am told, "just like pressing the start button on a furnace." In retrospect, it seems as if the true purpose of the block—can this be true?—is to provide experience giving such blocks, a standard procedure during childbirth, for the first year residents. Eagerly, they line up to insert the needle into my spine, and it is only after four have tried and failed that the attending physician steps in. Neither this block, nor any of the ones that follow, make any difference beyond a spectacularly bruised back.

"MS?" says the next doctor, the one in private practice who combines homeopathic remedies with traditional medicine, the one who does not accept insurance. "I don't know what this is," he says, "but it certainly isn't MS. More like a sports injury. You've aggravated your connective tissue to the point where your immune system doesn't know when to quit."

It is true that I played the piano for four to five hours every day, dreaming of becoming a concert pianist despite "chronic tendinitis" in my arms and wrists. It is true that I walked and jogged with "shin splints" in my legs. A sports injury doesn't seem too far fetched. I try the special diet that the homeopathic doctor suggests, avoiding eggs, wheat, sugar, corn, dairy products, nuts. I swallow aloe vera juice, burdock root, goldenseal. I have cranial sacral therapy; I visit a chiropractor; I see an herbal healer who reads my irises and studies my tongue and prescribes several foul-smelling tinctures. When none of this works, I fly to Boston, to the sports medicine specialist I'd seen the previous fall. There, I have surgery on both legs to relieve raised pressure in the muscle compartments, but this leaves me even worse off than before, for not only do the incisions create more inflammation, but they result in permanent nerve damage that will complicate future diagnoses.

I fly home.

Three months pass as I wait for an opening at the Mayo Clinic in Rochester, Minnesota. It is here, in the fall of 1986, that I receive the first round of steroid therapy that appears to help: injections of cortisone, oral prednisone.

After that, my mother and I make the seven-hour drive to Rochester every six weeks. The clinic is a vast medical complex like something out of Kafka, complete with towers of paperwork, dimly lit waiting rooms, beeping machines, and inexplicable procedures. Shuttle buses run between the local motels and the main entrance to the clinic, where wheelchairs are stacked like shopping carts. My mother has learned to test a few, checking for stuck brakes and speed wobbles, before choosing the one she will use to push me to appointments and tests and follow-up appointments, stopping now and then to consult the map we've been issued along with my patient ID. Tiled halls lead to elevators that open onto tiled halls. Underground tunnels connect the clinics, crowded with people wearing the uniform mask of exhaustion: families in street clothes, doctors in scrubs, outpatients glancing at watches and maps, inpatients on stretchers, or pushing their own IVs. There are subterraneous boutiques, wig shops and flower shops, beauty parlors, restaurants. Balloons bubble out of doorways, bright colors jaundiced by fluorescent lights. Small battery-powered dogs—the year's impulse buy—shudder and yap in the display windows. When the corridor bends, fish-eye mirrors mounted near the ceiling let you see who or what is racing toward you—an EMT team, a power wheelchair, a defibrillation unit with BE CALM painted on its side.

At each appointment, I leave the wheelchair behind in the waiting room, crutching more and more slowly after the nurse, who assures me we're almost there, it isn't much further, or do I want my mother to bring me the wheelchair? I do not. It is desperately important that I meet each new doctor, each new technician or nurse, standing up—or, at least, sitting in a regular chair and not a clinic wheelchair. I want to prove that I'm not like the others, the sick, the hurt, the hopeless. Nope, not me, I'm different, I'm fun. One look at me and the doctor will see, must see, that this is some kind of mistake, that I'm really not like this at all.

But the truth is that my body is just one more mystery to be solved. Already, there are patients piling up in the waiting rooms. Appointment schedules have fallen behind. There are medical students who must be instructed, who stand in a weary half circle around the examining table as a nurse moves my crutches aside. The doctor may or may not look me in the eye, may or may not speak my name. Once again, I recite my medical history, the story that has swallowed all the others I might tell, a story that stretches out in front of me like the map my mother unfolds before pushing me off to my next appointment, an arrow pointing to YOU ARE HERE, a circle that represents the place I must go. There are halls and doorways, elevators and waiting rooms. The walls are painted in gentle pastels that are neither blue nor green, but something that is neither, indescribable, in between.

And then, after the last appointment, the new prescriptions, the cortisone injections, after the final restless night at the motel, there's the seven-hour drive back home. Mostly, the landscape does not change: bare-knuckled trees and barbed-wire fences, skeletal clouds drifting across an endless sky. Snow squalls pass like identical seasons, and sometimes we pull over to wait them out, and sometimes we do not. In the distance, we see dairy farms, Holsteins picking their way across frozen muck. A dog, coated in ice, lying dead in the median. A white cross hung with plastic flowers that have faded from red to fingernail pink. My mother fills the air with words as if she believes the right ones, the right combination, can somehow put everything right. I myself say less and less on these trips; I am exhausted, numb. But if I think, *My stomach hurts,* my mother's hand pats her purse for the Saltines. If I need to use the bathroom, my mother says, "I think there's a McDonald's coming up."

At the McDonald's, my mother pulls up to the side entrance. On bad days, she gets the wheelchair out of the trunk. On good days, she holds the door while I crutch the seven steps inside. There, I sink into the closest seat to rest while she goes back out to park the car. It's another ten or so steps to the bathroom and, once inside, another five steps to the closest stall. Then another fifteen-odd steps back to the table, where I wait while my mother gets herself a cup of coffee. I've come to love McDonald's, its regulated access, its reliable terrain. McDonald's, an oasis of certainty, where there's never a step to get inside, where I know the rest room doors will be wide enough for a wheelchair to pass, the stall big enough so I don't have to pee with the door open wide to accommodate the chair.

Today is a postcortisone day, a good day, and so I decide to crutch in. While my mother goes around the corner to place her order, I continue my Frankenstein lurch toward the nearest open table, telling myself not to be paranoid, nobody is staring, and so what if they are, so you're on crutches, so who cares? The stares are less furtive than the ones I get when I'm in the wheelchair, when people run their gaze over my legs, then quickly glance away.

Scoping for parts, my brother calls it.

"My goodness, what happened to you?" A woman with three young children sits in a nearby booth. "Were you in an accident or something?"

I shake my head, keep going. These are the questions I've grown to hate, even without suspecting, yet, that they'll follow me for the rest of my life like a complicated name, an alias I must live by. *What's wrong with you, what happened to you, what's the matter?* Sometimes they're prefaced with, *Do you mind if I ask you a personal question?* Often they're followed by a long account of another person's health complaint: an accident, a bout of cancer, a recent diagnosis.

I take another step, another. The children stare, following their mother's example.

"What happened?" she repeats. "Did you break your legs?"

I sit down facing the opposite direction, expressionless, pretending I haven't heard. There are two kinds of pain: the kind that can be protected—the lump in the breast, the loved one's death, the broken heart—and the other kind, the visible kind, the kind that, in my case, is the first thing people see. It's right there, out in the open, where anyone might choose to poke at it, probe it, satisfy their grim curiosity.

"What's wrong with that lady?" one of the children asks.

"Nothing a smile wouldn't cure," the woman says, in a voice I am meant to hear.

Hope is Dickinson's "thing with feathers," that transcendent little bird. It is also, as a doctor once pointed out to me, the very last thing in Pandora's box.

Immediately after every appointment, after each new round of injections, I get an emotional second wind. I decide I am going to get well, right now, no more messing around. I give myself pep talks. So my doctor believes I have systematic tendinitis caused by an overaggressive immune system? Well, cortisone suppresses the immune system; therefore, it is logical, it is *inevitable,* that the cortisone shots will work. I begin each day with positive affirmations. My doctor has described my tendinitis as a raging fire that must be contained, and so I imagine tall flames doused with cool water, sputtering out. I visualize myself healthy again, jogging on a beach, hiking down a wooded trail. Instead of watching TV, I discipline myself, make tapes of my school assignments, dictate papers to my mother. I write awful, earnest haiku with titles like "The Moon." I listen to Spanish language tapes, review my high school German. I phone the friends I haven't heard from and leave funny, upbeat messages on their answering machines.

But as the days pass, and the cortisone wears off, I find that once again, I am weaker, stiffer, more inflamed. It's harder to get up in the morning, harder to move around the house, harder to make myself eat. Desperate little thoughts flicker at the edge of my steely attitude, and soon I am doubting once more, I am thinking, *Is this never going to end?* Thinking, *What if I never get better?* Thinking, *What am I going to do?* I consider suicide, but I can't decide which would be worse—to cause my parents such terrible pain? Or to burden them with caring for me for the rest of my life?

My doctor asks: Is it really that I'm in *more* pain, or am I simply not tolerating pain as well?

I do not know. I cannot tell. My body does not seem to belong to me. That's fine. I leave it behind whenever I can:

through sleep, through daydreams, through a drifting, hazy vacantness.

My doctor recommends higher dosages of anti-inflammatories, orthotics, patience. Leg lifts and toe curls. Riding a stationary bike. Walking in a swimming pool. Only now I'm unable to stay upright in water. I'm unable to complete more than a few full revolutions on the bicycle. The pain leaves me thick-headed, motionless, silent. I cannot sleep, and yet, I feel as if I'm never fully awake.

In March 1987, he refers me to a pain management center in a separate wing of the clinic. There are pictures of Jonathan Livingston Seagull on the walls. There are rhyming poems illustrated with rainbows. People sit in a circle and talk about ways in which pain is merely an excuse for not living fully. If you want to move beyond pain, you must make a commitment to life! At the end of the meeting, everybody joins hands and admits they have no control over their pain, over anything. They bow their heads and turn themselves over to their Higher Power.

I say, Uh, just so I'm clear. You're empowering yourselves by . . . deciding that you're *powerless?*

The man to my left, whose hand I'd rather not be holding, assures me that it will all make sense after a while. I have no doubt this is true, for the pain management center believes in "total immersion therapy," and these people have been living here for three weeks with no mail, no phone calls, no outside contact. Such things are deemed "privileges," and they must be earned by reaching "set goals": giving up a wheelchair or cane, cutting back on medication. The man whose hand I'd rather not be holding has had chronic back pain ever since a fall. His face is ashen with the effort of sitting in his chair.

I tell my doctor the pain management center is not for me. He does not seem surprised. When he rubs his hands over his face, I believe he is nearly as frustrated as I am. I like him because, unlike other doctors I've seen, he isn't trying to avoid me or get rid of me, which is what most doctors do when it becomes clear that a patient isn't getting better. He is practical, helpful, considerate. Other doctors have noted how I struggle to pull up my foot after taking each step, a condition noted in my chart as "dropped" feet. This doctor promptly prescribes a leg brace that fits into my shoe and keeps my foot at ninety-degree angle. It's a small thing, but it removes my fear of tripping when I crutch, and I'm in a position to be grateful for small things.

"Let's try one more round of cortisone," he says.

The nurse swabs bright orange antiseptic on my ankles, on the inside of my legs, just above the knee, on my wrists. She tries to make me lie back on the table, but my doctor knows better by now, knows that I have to watch the needle, keep some semblance of control. He counts backward with me as the cortisone goes in, a feeling of impossible pressure, a surge of heaviness pushing outward from within the points of my body that hurt most of all. And, afterward, warmth. And relief that it's over.

"Come back in six weeks," he says. "If you're still not responding, we'll talk about other options."

Other options: I have no idea what this means. But whatever these options are, I will take them, I'll obey, I'll be the model patient—not like I used to be.

Home again, I can't stop thinking about the years leading up to my first medical leave: what I should have done, what I might have done, how I might have prevented all this from happening. If I'd taken a medical leave after my first year at the Peabody Conservatory, if I'd given myself even a month away from the piano, might that have made a difference in my hands? If I'd stopped jogging with friends, would my legs have healed by now? What if, after leaving the Conservatory, I'd gone home to my parents right away instead of staying out east the way I did, working in Connecticut, Florida, Maine, scrambling to make ends meet? What if I hadn't enrolled at the University of Maine, if I'd let college slide for a while? If I'd seen better doctors when I'd first started to limp? If I'd used my crutches consistently instead of cheating, forgetting to bring them with me, finding reasons to leave them home?

I think about how there was a time in my life when I believed that having to give up the piano was the worst thing that could ever happen to me. I think about the Conservatory, and my friends there, and the rhythms of my old life. I think about the new life I'd tried to make for myself in Maine. I joined a bird-watchers' club, but could not keep up on the hikes. I enrolled in an evening dance class, flung myself around, told myself not to be such a baby, nothing could possibly hurt this much. The pain, I told myself, *had* to be all in my head. I *would* get on top of it by sheer force of will. Then, one night, I was truly afraid I might not make it home. I stopped to rest on benches, on retaining walls, coaching myself along: *three more blocks, c'mon, just a little further.*

The first campus doctor I saw prescribed the same anti-inflammatories that the doctors at the Conservatory had recommended. These anti-inflammatories had given me gastrointestinal problems when I'd taken them before, but the campus doctor said I'd have to deal with it, it couldn't be helped. He also prescribed vitamins. I was, he said, "shockingly" weak. How long had it been since I'd stopped exercising? This, he told me sternly, was only making my problems worse. It was important to keep moving, to do low-impact exercises, to swim at the university pool. When he heard that I'd spent my childhood at the piano, the past two years in a conservatory practice room, he'd shaken his head. "We've got to get you in shape, young lady," he said. "Your ankles are so weak that I don't see how you can stand."

He gave me a pair of crutches, demonstrated how he wanted me to use them. The prescription was for three weeks.

I forced myself to crutch briskly to the end of the block, then sat on the curb, arms and legs burning. It seemed as if a week couldn't pass without the realization that there was yet another thing I couldn't do without pain: hurry across the street as the light changed, climb stairs, walk between classes without stopping, keep up taking notes. The anti-inflammatories smoldered in my stomach. Nights, I lay awake thinking, *What the hell is the matter with me?* Thinking, *I can't believe this is happening.* Thinking, *I must be losing my mind.*

There is a period of time, after someone falls ill, when the world is acutely sympathetic. Friends visit, acquaintances phone; co-workers not only offer to help, but sometimes, they actually do. People collect anecdotes about others who have overcome illness and misfortune and present them to you like spectacular bouquets: hopefully, nervously, sincerely. They are evidence that your own troubles are not insurmountable. They are proof that it's only a matter of time before you, too, will be back on your feet. Your sickroom grows thick with these invisible flowers. You inhale their strange perfume. You study their untarnished petals, their pure colors, and you notice that, like artificial flowers, they are too neat, too orderly. Each is the exact same size and shape. Each is too regular to be real.

These anecdotes follow the Aristotelian model of storytelling, the one you had to memorize in high school, the one to which every work of fiction you discussed got strapped, howling, like a martyr to a rack. Each begins with an *inciting incident:* a mysterious seizure, a freak accident, an inexplicable symptom. This is followed by *rising action:* the trip to the emergency room, visits to specialists, moments of doubt and despair. Finally, there is a *climax:* the surgery or treatment, everything touch and go. If there is a supernatural element to this anecdote, it's likely to appear at this point: a tunnel of light, the voice of God, the appearance of an angel. And at last, comes the *denouement:* a resolution, a cure or, failing that, a clear prognosis, a lesson learned.

But what if your story shapes itself differently? What if there is no climax, no resolution, only the passing days, the paralyzing uncertainty, the gradually dawning sense that, regardless of what happens next, you will never return to the country you have left, to the body you once took for granted? What if things simply happen because they do, and then you pick yourself up, or not? What kind of story is that?

When an old friend from the Conservatory flies in for the weekend, she takes one look at me and says, *Oh, my god,* before she can stop herself. Both of us laugh, but soon the conversation thins. I am unable to do the things that formed the backbone of our friendship—going out, going dancing, going shopping, going to the gym. *Going*. We met the day we moved into the dorms and for two years, we saw each other every day, studied together, performed together, spent vacations with each other's families. Even after I left, we spoke on the phone, mailed each other silly photo-essays of our lives, shared spring breaks in cities like New York and Washington, D.C.

During the fifteen months I've been home, inert, Susan has kept moving. She is auditioning for graduate schools. She has two lovers, each a secret from the other. She keeps asking, What are you going to *do*? She is the daughter of a psychiatrist, and she says that if there was really something wrong with me, something *organically* wrong with me, the doctors would have figured it out by now—wouldn't they? A minute later, she's telling me about somebody who died of cancer only months after the family doctor had dismissed her with a prescription for Valium. Maybe I should come out east again. Maybe her father could recommend a diagnostician, a neurologist, a rheumatoid specialist.

"I'm at one of the best clinics in the country," I say. "I've already seen every kind of doctor."

Susan rages. She shines with indignation on my behalf. How can this be *happening*? She paces the bedroom, runs her hands through her pretty, cropped hair. I try to keep up, to pay attention, but pain makes it hard to concentrate.

"What?" I say, and she says angrily, "You aren't even listening to me!"

On the second day, we go to a movie. She has to load the clattering wheelchair in and out of my mother's car, and we both pretend it's perfectly natural for her to be driving that car instead of me. She has to push me into the theater, sit with me in a folding chair behind the last row of seats, where the manager makes us sit because of "fire regulations." A group of teenaged boys, not much younger than we are, are already seated nearby. They stare at me, then at Susan; they whisper among themselves. As soon as the lights go down, they begin, in falsetto:

"*Je*-sus, heal me!"

"O, *Lawd,* help me *WALK* again!"

One of them asks the others in a loud, clear voice: "How do you eat a vegetable?" But I already know the punch line: "Crawl under the wheelchair." These boys, it seems, are everywhere, like Dutch Elm disease, like mosquitoes. They make jokes, talk in falsetto. They roll down their windows to shout things as they drive past in their cars; they holler from fraternity porches, *Hey, sexy! Yeah, you! Got a boyfriend?*

We leave the theater early, drive home. Susan helps me into the house. That night, in the double bed we've shared comfortably and easily during past visits, she hugs the edge, keeping even the warmth of her body from touching my own. Or maybe it's me who has become so distant I cannot feel her near me. A few months later, she phones to let me know she's been accepted at a graduate school in Chicago, just a few hours away.

"It'll be great!" she says. "I can come up and see you."

But she doesn't send me her new address, doesn't reply to the letters I send to her over the summer in care of her parents' address. It takes a while before I understand I'll never see her again.

In April 1987, when I phone my doctor for our scheduled consultation, I tell him that things are still getting worse. That I'm weaker, more inflamed. My doctor does not seem surprised, and I sense that something has changed. Usually, he voices my own frustration, my own disappointment, then urges me not to worry. These things can be stubborn, he says. He assures me that he's seen worse. But this time, after a careful pause, he tells me he has discussed my case with a new doctor, a neurologist I haven't yet seen. This neurologist would like to meet with me as soon as possible. This neurologist will be coordinating my case from now on. This neurologist feels the abnormalities in my nerve conduction studies are not a result of surgical damage, but a systematic muscle disorder of some kind. He has reviewed my last MRI and would like me to have another. It is obvious that the current treatment isn't working.

The time for *other options* has arrived.

"So—if the cortisone hasn't worked . . ." I say. I have learned that if you pitch your voice low, it is nearly impossible to cry. "I mean, I'm almost twenty-three and I still don't know—"

He's a doctor who does not interrupt.

"I just don't know how I'm going to wait any longer," I finally say.

My doctor says he agrees, that there really is no point in waiting anymore. It could be years before I have a firm diagnosis. It is time to think about a motorized wheelchair or scooter, something I can use independently. He'll set me up for an evaluation to decide what will work best.

"Ultimately, it's your decision," my doctor says. "But I think we have to look in this direction. Get you moving again, get you back in school."

A thought forms itself in my mind, floats there like a dust mote, detached. *So this, then, is what my life will be.*

We schedule an appointment for the following week.

One of my uncles used a wheelchair, a result of complications from diabetes. He was a smart, funny, opinionated man, an avid fly-fisherman, an accomplished amateur photographer. He and my aunt and their children were always doing interesting things: visiting national parks and historic sites, camping, canoeing. In my family, "vacation" meant a long weekend at a Holiday Inn, my brother and I circling our mother in the pool like frenzied sharks, shrieking, "Mom, look at this! Watch me!" while our father napped in the room. But my uncle's family was different. He, like my aunt, had a college degree. They owned things like binoculars and wildlife guides. They built camp fires and made s'mores, and if they caught a fish that was too small, they actually threw it back, the way you were supposed to, instead of smacking its head on a rock so that you wouldn't wind up catching it again.

One day, when I was eight or nine, the subject of my uncle's wheelchair came up among a few of my older cousins. They were smoking pin joints in the orchard, passing a can of beer back and forth as we younger ones looked on with love and longing.

"If I had to be in a wheelchair," one of them said, "I'd kill myself."

And all of us agreed.

Alone in my room, I stare at the folding wheelchair we've been renting. At my crutches, at my leg braces, which my mother calls my "ducks," leaning up against the closet door. At the wobbly card table. The electric typewriter. A few battered paperbacks from the library that I don't read because holding them open, turning the pages, inflames my arms and hands. Even now, after all this time, there's a part of me that fully expects to wake up one morning and find myself healed. To walk out of this house and back into my life as if nothing has changed. A part of me is still waiting for a clear diagnosis, a prognosis, a plan. But I could wait here forever, hoping for that story and all its validations. Seeking a reason, an answer, the climax, as my life shrinks to fit the confines of this room. My body shrinking, too, growing passive, lighter, empty.

I think of something my father told me: how, at six-foot-one, his weight had fallen to 125 pounds by the time he entered the san.

"What did you do?" I asked, unable to imagine him that thin.

"What did I do," he repeated. He was standing in the doorway, his shoulders bristling with light; he raised his hands. "What did I do." Then, abruptly, he laughed.

"I stayed out of the wind," he said.

I am learning a technique I will rely on when I start to write fiction. I am exploring one thing by looking at another. Describing the absent landscape that defines my subject's shape. The brightness of the light from the hallway that outlines my father's outstretched hands.

Three

My mother could turn anything into a story. Nights, when she tucked me into bed, she'd ask me what color kiss I wanted, then wait while I tried to describe what I saw. A red kiss, bright as a zinnia. A fat, orange kiss, like the fish in its bowl. Earthworm kisses that tickled and twisted, slid down the back of your neck. "What color kiss tonight?" she'd say, after listening to my prayers, and I'd try to come up with something new, a color I'd never tried before. A kiss the color of the palm of my hand. A kiss the color of my grandmother's hair. My favorite kiss was exactly the color of the sky before a storm, smoky blue with purple streaks along the horizon, but this kiss took a lot of time and my mother could only deliver one if her papers were all graded and her lesson plans finished and the housework reasonably under control. Then she'd wrap me tight in the blankets, roll me to and fro like the wind, lift me up and drop me like thunder on the bed. The rain was her fingers up and down my back. The purple came afterward, the pressure of her hand on my forehead. And then a blue whisper over my hair, soothing, smoothing, stroking the clouds away.

At the piano, my mother spoke not of sound but color, not of notes but what the chords might stand for, what they made me feel. My brother preferred to sit under the piano, working the pedals with his hands, while my mother and I sat together on the bench, telling stories on the shining keys. Perhaps she picked out a swervy melody as I knuckled the black keys into frenzy. Or we might take turns mashing the white keys with the palms of our hands, a line of broad, flat stones. Sometimes I'd choose a song from one of her old music books: "Spinning Song" or "Tarantella" or selections from *The King and I.*

"Play this one," I'd say, pointing to a measure. "Play this one." And I'd play back what I heard.

When I was seven, I started formal lessons. My first assignment was a series of rhythmic variations on "Twinkle, Twinkle, Little Star." The most difficult one went *da*-da-da-da, *da*-da-da-da—Think of *rutabaga, rutabaga,* my teacher said—and when I finished, my wrists ached all the way up my arms. I remember my surprise. I'd never guessed, watching my mother, that playing the piano *hurt.*

"Shake it out," my teacher told me in her lovely alto voice. "Thatta girl. Shake it all out."

I rode my bike home through a canopy of elm trees, weaving between the puddles of sunlight scattered across the sidewalks. That night at the piano, my mother listened to what I'd learned.

"The rutabagas hurt me," I explained, holding out my hands. My mother cupped them in her own, studied them very seriously. Then she covered them with kisses the cold, clear color of ice.

In my family, no one complained about a cut, a bump, a bruise. "Anything broken?" the nearest adult would say if you tripped and fell. "No? Then what are you crying for?"

Illness was something to be hidden. If it was discovered, you still went to school or to work, of course, but when you got home you were quarantined in your room, so whatever you had wouldn't spread. All it took was a sneeze to rouse my father's suspicions. "You catching *schnupe?*" he'd say. My brother and I would deny it fiercely—who wanted to be isolated from the family room TV? At school, kids ran the water fountain twice, to kill the germs, before taking a drink; in the bathrooms, we put toilet paper on the seats before we sat, the way that our parents had taught us, so we wouldn't catch some sex disease. Cleanliness was next to godliness. The moment we got home, we washed our hands with hot water and soap. We washed them again before meals, and one last time before bed. You just couldn't be too careful.

Ringworm, on the other hand, wasn't so serious. Everybody had that. You just soaked a couple of Band-Aids in kerosene, plastered them on, and left them there as long as you could stand it.

Pinworms passed with enough castor oil; pinkeye with saltwater flushes.

Doctoring people wasn't much different than doctoring livestock, and anyone could do that.

Sore throat? Take a hydrogen peroxide gargle.

Head cold? Hot whiskey punch with lemon and sugar.

Fever? Ice bath, if it got high enough. Otherwise, drink lots of water and for Chrissake sake, don't eat *anything*.

Toothache? Chew on the other side of your mouth and see if it don't get better.

Earache? Lie on a warm heating pad, or else ask Uncle Artie to blow a little warm cigar smoke in there.

Sprain something? Well, don't step on it, silly. Keep your mind off it, keep busy, forget about it. At night, make up a plastic bag of ice, wrap it in a towel, and take it to bed.

Headache? "Stick your head in the toilet for ten minutes," my father would tease. "I guarantee you won't feel a thing after that."

There was no such thing as mental illness. There was *craziness,* of course, but there really wasn't any cure for that. *Character flaws* such as moodiness or laziness could be easily relieved by doing something nice for somebody else, getting your mind off yourself, thinking about those less fortunate. A smile's just a frown turned upside down. Nobody saw a psychiatrist, except on TV.

My mother accidentally dislocated my shoulder once while she was playing with me, swinging me in circles by my outstretched arms. When I cried, she scolded me for acting like a baby—my arm looked fine, there was nothing the matter with me. Alone in my room, I felt it pop back into place, but then it swelled, and we wound up at the emergency room. By then, my mother was beside herself, but when the X rays came back, we were both a little embarrassed. We could have saved ourselves the trouble, the expense. A couple of days on the heating pad, the way my father had suggested, and it would have been fine.

Several years later, when I knocked myself unconscious practicing gymnastic flips, the first thing I did after coming to was beg the other kids not to tell. Around that time, my mother, on a dare, ran the school's annual thousand-yard dash alongside her students. The next day she was hospitalized; she'd had pneumonia, it turned out, for nearly a week.

"I'd been feeling really lousy," she admitted. "I thought it was just me."

Cancer, on the other hand, you didn't mess around with. If you found a lump, you didn't tell a soul. You didn't even say a word like that outright. Nobody knew exactly how you caught it, so if somebody's mother or father had cancer, you weren't allowed play at their house, though you could play in their yard where there was plenty of fresh air.

This was rural Wisconsin in the 1970s. Farmers, and the children of farmers. Germans and Luxemburgers and Czechs, Italians who'd worked in the local quarries at the turn of the century. Dutch who drove cars that sported bumper stickers boasting IF YOU AIN'T DUTCH, YOU AIN'T MUCH. No blacks. No Jews. A few families from the Philippines. Everybody knew who was what. It was the second, question you asked at school, right after *What church do you go to?*

At my elementary school class graduation, awards were given for Best Attendance. I coveted that prize, but my best friend, Tabitha, won. She'd come to school despite strep throat, several colds, the stomach flu (though she'd been confined to the nurse's office), and a case of chicken pox cleverly concealed beneath a turtleneck sweater.

My parents grew up on dairy farms less than ten miles apart, the grandchildren of Luxemburg and German immigrants. At sixteen, my father left high school to farm full time with my grandfather, and it was common, in good weather, for the two of them to work sixteen-hour days. After marrying my mother, my father threw that same energy into selling fertilizer and, later, farm machinery, traveling for the Gehl corporation on marathon routes throughout the Midwest, saving money to start his own company. He came home every weekend, but he was something of a stranger, distant, unfamiliar with our household routines. Saturdays, he worked at his desk in the family room, going over ledgers as the adding machine chimed its toneless song. Sunday nights, before he went back on the road, he spread newspapers over the family room carpet and polished his wingtips with an old diaper. My brother and I watched, curious but shy, inhaling the deep sweet smell of the polish. If we asked whose diaper it had been, my father sometimes said, *Ann Manette's,* calling me by my full name, the name of my childhood. Other times he'd say, *Michael's.* This lack of consistency both fascinated and frightened us, for our mother was exacting in her answers, no matter how foolish our questions, and no matter how many times we asked.

Mostly, on those weekends my father was home, my mother kept us occupied with projects in the kitchen, away from his desk, away from his briefcase with its tempting, snapping locks. Or she took us out to her mother's farm where, likely as not, there'd be a handful of cousins and second cousins swarming the rusty swing set by the chicken coop, a couple of aunts plus a distant relation or two playing Scrabble in the kitchen, uncles watching TV in the living room. Grandma Krier not only welcomed us; she expected us. A weekend with less than a dozen visitors was considered a lonely weekend indeed. And you always showed up with room in your stomach—there was no point in protesting that you'd just eaten.

Grandma Krier's cavernous refrigerator was crowded with bottles and tins, stacks of wrapped platters, Tupperware containers of all sizes, mysterious lumps of foil, soft cheeses, bean salads, jars of raw whole milk with the cream thick at the top, and—in summer—zucchini breads and cakes, not to mention raw zucchinis, which always seemed to multiply in the crisper. A pungent, not wholly unpleasant odor rose from the racks when you opened the refrigerator door. Sometimes, my mother would have me lure my grandmother out of the house, and then she'd sneak into the kitchen and throw out what she called *the questionables.* The basement root cellar was overflowing as well, the bins filled with onions, apples, pears, potatoes with sprouts as long as my arms. Once, on a shelf behind the old wringer-style washer, I found a box of murky preserves dated 1955.

For years, Grandma Krier worked as head cook at the

community center in Belgium, supervising wedding suppers and graduation banquets, funeral receptions and family reunion brunches. Before that, she'd cooked for her family of nine children, plus whichever of the "city cousins"—an assortment of relatives from Milwaukee—happened to be visiting. Summers, these numbers swelled further with the "trashers," threshing crews made up of local farmers who took turns working one another's fields, cultivating in spring, bringing in the harvest at summer's end.

"I don't cook small," she'd say, "because it just looks wrong in the pan."

My mother was the baby of the family, the youngest of seven sisters and a much awaited brother who'd arrived next-to-last—*just as we'd given up hope,* according to family lore. All had married and were busy raising children of their own within a twenty-mile radius of my grandmother's farm. I had sixty-odd cousins and over a hundred second cousins, and it seemed that I saw at least a third of them every weekend on the farm. When the house got too full, we kids were sent out to the barn. Winters, we played hide-and-seek on the upper level where the heavy machinery was stored, or else we climbed the ladder to the hay mow, where we swung on the rope swing, or hunted for mouse nests, or stacked hay bales into spectacular, multiroomed forts. Outside, we sledded on my grandmother's dead-end road, which had two hills: one good, one better. Summers, we moved out into the surrounding fields, building forbidden forts in the corn, hunting for arrowheads between the rows of soybeans. We picked cherries and mulberries, asparagus and rhubarb, and when the spray-trucks came by to douse the apple orchard with pesticide, we concealed ourselves in the branches, weathering each blast, a game we called *Hurricane*. On rainy days, we set up dominoes in the sour-smelling milk house, played crazy eights or slapjack beneath the shelter of the porch awning. My grandmother would have happily provided us with a midafternoon snack, but my brother and I preferred to sneak into the basement through the root cellar door and raid the apple bin, the pantry—just as our mother had done.

Our mother had loved farming as much as our father had hated it. (In junior high, when I asked for horseback-riding lessons, he refused, saying, "Don't you see I work like I do so you won't ever need to mess with things like that?") Though she'd graduated from a Catholic women's college, and now taught fifth grade, her arms were still thickly muscled from fieldwork, her shoulders broad from lugging buckets of milk, bales of hay, sacks of feed. Her father, my Grandpa Krier, had died in a farming accident when she was two, and my grandmother had managed to keep the family's one hundred acres intact with only the help of her children, plus a hired man named Irwin. Summers, Irwin preferred the barn to his room in the house, and, at night, my mother and her sisters watched him from an upstairs window, following the glow of his cigarette as he passed in front of the open barn door. He liked to go out for a drink once in a while. He put ketchup on everything, from eggs to bread. His cigarette butt smoking on a nearby saucer. His cough like a private language.

"But when was his birthday?" I asked my mother, pressing for more, always more. Irwin had died of emphysema the year before I was born.

"I don't know," my mother said, but I wouldn't accept this, couldn't. At ten, I still believed my mother knew everything. It was a belief I'd cherished, protected, long after I'd stalked and killed the Easter bunny, the tooth fairy, Saint Nicholas.

"What was his favorite color?" I demanded. "What was his middle name?"

"I've already told you everything I know," my mother said, evenly. "Sweetheart, he's been dead for over ten years."

One day, I begged her to make up the answers, and when she refused, I stomped up the stairs to my room and slammed the door so hard that the framed needlepoints fell off the wall. I'd always assumed that every question, large or small, would have its corresponding answer. But Irwin was, and would remain, an open-ended question, a mystery my mother refused to illuminate with a lie. Lying was a sin.

Telling stories that weren't true, even if everybody *knew* they weren't true, was the same thing, only said differently. There was right and there was wrong. There was good and there was bad. Mine was a world of black and white; there was nothing in between.

I believe there is a relationship, much like that between parent and child, between the physical, or external, landscape we call *home* and the spiritual, or internal, landscape that becomes the human soul. I was the offspring of manicured lawns, of perfectly rectangular ranch houses laid out on perfectly rectangular lots, of streets that met at right angles. Following directions, there was never any question which way was left, which way right, which way straight ahead. The roads leading out of town parted the flat fields neatly, cutting more rectangles, precise as stained glass: gold and green in the summertime; white and dun in winter, black when the land was freshly cultivated, speckled with seagulls like smooth, gray stones. Lake Michigan edged the horizon like the bright, blue border on a quilt. *A place for everything; everything in its place,* I was told, and the landscape bore witness to those words. You could see the truth of it laid out for miles. Faith was clean-cut as a corn row or a fence line, direct as a county highway. God was the hawk, high overhead, overlooking us all. We were the rabbits, trying to blend in, trying not to draw attention to ourselves.

This is just the way things are. If you don't like it, take it up with God.

Summers, restless, I'd get on my bike and ride out of town as far as I could. After an hour or so, I'd coast to a stop and wait for the lake breeze to cool me. Around me, the fields would be planted in soybeans, field corn and sweet corn, oats, wheat. In the distance there'd be a little white farmhouse beside a red barn, a windmill in the courtyard slowly turning. Perhaps I'd see a herd of Holsteins taking their shade beneath a single stand of hickory trees. A frenzy of black-eyed susans in the run-off ditches. An orange housecat, bright as a button, stalking something in the weeds. After catching my breath, I'd get back on my bike and, again, I'd ride and ride until my hot breath burned my upper lip and the pavement seemed to rise and fall with each pump of my knees. At last, I'd coast to a stop, look around . . .

. . . and the fields would be planted in soybeans, field corn and sweet corn, oats, wheat. Once again, there'd be that little white farmhouse beside its red barn, a windmill in the courtyard slowly turning. Another herd of Holsteins, larger perhaps. A meadow lark balancing on a telephone line. A ragged cluster of purple-headed thistles, day lilies rising around it in a fiery cloud.

This was not a landscape that encouraged individual interpretations, diverse opinions, conflict. The Catholic

God we worshipped was a God who did not permit negotiations, a God who came and went like the seasons, a God who moved in mysterious ways. There was no mention of anything like *a personal relationship with Christ.* There were rules, there were beliefs, and you could like them or lump them but you had to obey. The madder you got, the harder you smiled.

If you can't say something nice, don't say anything at all.

You did what you were told. You believed what you were taught. *Dear Senator,* I wrote with the other members of my catechism class. *Please stop the murder of helpless unborn babies. Dear Senator, Homosexuality is a perversion of God's most sacred laws.*

Dear Senator. Dear God. It terrifies me, now. I would have written anything, believed anything. Absolutely anything at all.

God was Love, yes, but the icy stream that fed this love was Fear. When storms blew in off Lake Michigan, turning the sky an almost supernatural green, where did the lightning strike? Not the fields or the roads. Not the low-lying houses and milk sheds, the chicken coops and corn cribs. No, it struck the windmills, the power lines, the stands of hickory trees. It scorched whatever dared to stand up, stand out, stand alone.

"What should you do," my mother drilled my brother and me, "if you ever get caught out in the open during a storm?"

But we already knew the answer. It was something we learned in school.

Lie down. Keep still. Wait for the thunder to pass.

Each time I left Grandma Krier's house, she pressed her faith firmly into my hands, like lunch money, like a map should I ever get lost. Her Catholicism reflected the view she saw every day from her kitchen windows: few shadows. Straight lines. A precise, uncomplicated horizon.

Her name, until her marriage, was Margaret Catherine Jacoby; her birth certificate, which I learned of after her death, read *Margaretta Katarina Jacobi.* She loved to tell the story of how my grandfather's parents, who owned the adjacent farm, had carried him, a babe in arms, to the wedding of her mother and father. "We made the boy," they said. "Now you two make the girl."

And her mother and father did.

From the time she was born, in 1899, it was understood by everyone that my grandmother would grow up to marry Otto Krier. Even as children, they'd loved each other. My grandmother followed him everywhere, like an adoring younger sister. At school, my grandfather made sure the other boys included her in their games. When the first world war threatened overseas, and speaking anything but English was forbidden, they stood side by side in the schoolyard, scratching notes to each other in the dirt.

Neither of them knew English very well at that time; they spoke Luxemburg with their families, German with neighbors and friends. Both would end their formal educations after finishing eighth grade. There was too much work to be done at home. Advanced education was a luxury.

Grandma Krier was never one to voice regrets, but several times, when I was growing up, she said she wished she'd gone to high school. "So I would be smart," was how she put it, her tone flat, without self-pity. And yet, she'd continued to educate herself by reading the English dictionary, which she kept pushed to the center of the kitchen table, in easy reach. She also read the Bible, the newspaper, the almanac, in addition to a number of religious publications. She spoke and wrote Luxemburg and German, as well as English, and could carry on a conversation in Dutch. At ninety, she still beat nearly everyone at Scrabble. At ninety-five, furious, she phoned my mother with a list of words: *Internet, cyberspace, modem.* My mother defined them one by one, but my grandmother wasn't appeased. "They shouldn't be allowed to have words that aren't in the dictionary," she said.

I see her now as she pulls a steaming pan of chicken from the oven. She strides impatiently into the center of the thickest raspberry patch, ignoring the thorns that tug and tear at the loose skin on her arms. Winters, she walks out to the barn through the drifts wearing only a short-sleeved dress, ladies' shoes from J C Penney's, hose striped with runs. If one of the geese forgets itself and hisses, she snatches it up by the neck and swings it forward and back.

"Mind your manners," she says, then lets it sail.

She never raises her voice to her grandchildren. She doesn't have to. When my brother refuses to eat his liver and onions, she offers to fix him a ground glass sandwich instead. We know she isn't joking. My brother cleans his plate. I take a second helping, just to be safe.

My father calls her *Big Mama*—but never to her face.

Even the bull knows enough to leave her alone.

She tells us the story of *going to get her tonsils yanked.* It was 1908. Her father hitched the horses to the wagon and took her into "town," which would have meant Random Lake. A nurse held her mouth open as Doctor reached down her throat with a long-handled scissors. There was no anesthetic, not even a piece of ice to suck. Her father paid the bill, then drove her back home.

"Did you cry?" I want to know.

"What good would that have done?" she says, and she's right.

Sundays after Mass, we cross the street to the cemetery, where she tidies my grandfather's grave. I long to know more about his death, but my grandmother deflects my questions, pretends she doesn't hear. I have only the facts from my mother, who was too young to remember him, who knows no more than this: that he lost his balance and fell off a wagon, landing on a pitchfork. That he didn't die right away. That the night of his wake, the aurora borealis appeared, and no one could remember having ever seen it so bright. People believed it was my grandfather's message from heaven, his good-bye.

Walking back to the car, my grandmother spots a thistle growing in the lawn. Without warning, she jackknifes at the waist, jerks it up. "Toss this in the field," she says. I accept it like a crown of thorns. Her own hands are so callused that the prickers don't stick. She brushes them off like flour.

There is strength in my family, and then there is weakness.

My other grandmother, my father's mother, doesn't like me any better than she did when I was five, though she's awfully fond of my brother. My mother says I shouldn't take it personally. Grandma Ansay, she says, is *old-fashioned,* and *old-fashioned* people like boys better than girls. It isn't fair, but it can't be helped.

Grandma Ansay tries to wheedle my brother away from my mother whenever she can. Sometimes she pulls him aside and gives him a gift. It could be a quarter, or a brand-new watch, or a savings bond. By now, she's had *her stroke*—that's what we call it, as if it's something she's selected for herself, like a peculiar hat—and she walks with a cane, dragging one leg. Her speech is slurred. She often cries. But then, she's been sickly all her life, always complaining: this ache, that pain. My father doesn't call her Big Mama or Mom or Ma or anything else, although he says *Mother* when he's speaking about her in the third person, as in *Mother never came with us to the fields* and *Pa always said that Mother bought shoes to fit her head and not her feet.*

Twice a month, we have dinner at this grandmother's house. "Dinner" means a meal that is eaten at noon. Grandma Ansay keeps the thermostat set at eighty-five Her enema bottle hangs behind the bathroom door, and the house smells of Ben-Gay and a terrible, unnamed sadness. She pokes at my flat chest to see if I'm developing. She tries to look up my dress, then laughs when I slap it down.

At the dinner table, she and my grandfather bicker until Grandpa says, "That's enough out of you!" Then they fight in earnest, speaking their own venomous mix of Luxemburg, English, and German, while my mother and father and brother and I keep eating, as if nothing whatsoever is wrong. Please pass the peas. Please pass the bread. Nothing has changed since the brief time we lived with them.

"I'll tell them everything, if that's what you want," Grandpa finally says. "I'll tell them all about you!"

Tell us *what?* Personally, I am dying to know. I figure it must have to do with either sex or money, the Twin Taboos, the two things nice people never talk about. But Grandma's tongue is tired and cannot shape the words. She gives up, stops arguing. Instead, she stares at her hands, chained together by the rosary in her lap. After the meal, she lies face down on the daybed, weeping quietly, furiously. I watch her from the doorway. In catechism, our teacher—the mother of one of my friends—explains that if we only have faith the size of a mustard seed, God will work miracles in our lives and grant us any request. She even passes around a tiny yellowish husk, so we can see for ourselves that this isn't so much to ask. Then she tells us, in graphic detail, about her miscarriages, how everybody told her she'd never carry a child to term, but look—here's her daughter, Mary Elizabeth, who sits among us smiling like the Gift from God she is. We can reach out and touch Mary Elizabeth, the way Doubting Thomas touched Jesus. We can see for ourselves the power of faith.

I love my religion classes, which are held in our teacher's home. Mrs. T. always pulls the shades and lights tall, white candles. It's better than ghost stories at camp. We hold hands and chant Hail Marys. Once, as we're talking about Saint Benedict, we all see Satan circling us in the form of a small blue light. But because we're each wearing a Saint Benedict medal, blessed by the Pope himself, Satan can't do a thing to us and eventually the light winks out. That night, Mrs. T. holds a special ceremony in which we each vow to wear our medals until our deaths. I keep mine pinned to my underwear; when I shower, I hold it in my mouth. I will wear it until I'm in college. I'll have nightmares when I finally take it off.

Grandma Ansay prays all the time, but clearly, she's doing something wrong. Why else wouldn't God make her better? And why would God give her a stroke in the first place, if it wasn't something she deserved? At Mass on Sundays, we pray for the intentions of particular people who are sick, and some of them get better, and some of them don't. Either way, there must be a reason, and that reason is implied by every Bible story we read, every sermon that we hear. The good are rewarded. The bad are punished. When someone gets better and returns to church, everybody congratulates them, shakes their hands. When somebody doesn't get better, well, it's always a little bit awkward. The priest speaks of *mystery,* and we say the Our Father: *thy kingdom come, thy will be done.* God wants some people to suffer, like it or lump it, and He isn't saying why. But it isn't just luck. There is a Master Plan.

Certainly, no one who gets better ever thinks it's just dumb luck.

"Your grandmother used to sing, and play the organ. She loved to dance," my mother says. "Imagine how frustrating it would be if you couldn't do the things you loved."

But I don't imagine, because I know I'd never let something like that happen to me.

At twenty-one, on medical leave, I receive a letter from a

college friend. By now, mail seldom arrives for me, unless it contains a bill from a hospital or clinic. I take the letter from the kitchen, where my mother has handed it to me, and head toward the privacy of my bedroom. Crutching across the house leaves my arms and legs feeling as if the muscles are being pulled from the bone. It's winter, but I'm wearing shorts because the scrape of fabric is unbearable against my shins. My mother has strategically placed a dining room chair in the hall, and I decide to stop and read the letter here, instead of taking the next fifteen steps to my bedroom, just in case I need those steps to get to the bathroom later. My days are divided up this way, a sequence of bargains and rationings. Do I shower in the morning and then rest until lunch time, or do I shower in the evening, when I can go directly to bed afterward? If I answer the phone in the kitchen, will I be stranded for an hour, for an afternoon?

The letter is short. My friend is angry with me, disgusted. This is the last time she'll write.

"How can you let this happen to yourself?" she says.

I'm the second-fastest kid at Lincoln Elementary—only Jimmy Borganhagen, who can do three hundred sit-ups and seventy-five push-ups, can beat me. In my mind, his ability to do sit-ups and push-ups has married his unbelievable speed, and I start doing sit-ups before I say my bedtime prayers, boy sit-ups, my feet hooked beneath my bed. I do push-ups, too; I can even manage a clap in between. I eat lots of bananas, because I've heard this is what weight lifters do.

"Feel my muscle," I tell my brother, my mother, my best friend, Tabitha, who I wrestle to the ground every so often, just because I can. In the kitchen, while my mother is at work, my brother and I take turns mixing concoctions of vinegar, baking soda, pickle juice, chocolate syrup—the one who can't swallow the other's bitter medicine loses. We judge each other, our friends, our cousins by one standard: toughness. When Mike jumps off the hood of the car, I jump off its roof. When he does the same, I pull the ladder out of the garage, shimmy up the side of the house, and fling myself into the side yard, where the grass is longer, softer. Summer mornings, we both chase after the garbage truck on our bicycles, but I'm the one who gets close enough to high-five the sanitation worker's outstretched hand. "No fair," Mike says, and he's right. I'm two and a half years older. Taller. Stronger.

"That will change," my father says, but he's been saying that since the day my mother brought Mike home from the hospital, his head like an overripe tomato, wrapped in a brilliant blue blanket. I hated the way my father immediately started calling him Tiger. "Call *me* Tiger," I insisted, but my nickname was already Pumpkin, which I hated. Pumpkins weren't tough. Pumpkins got their guts carved out, then sat in people's windows, rotting slowly, their faces caving in on themselves.

I'm no pumpkin. At school, Bonnie Adelsky—a big girl with breasts, who has been held back—arranges a wrestling match between me and a junior high school boy. We meet behind the teacher's parking lot late in the afternoon. While he's busy protecting his balls—as if I cared—I throw myself at his ankles, and as soon as I've got him on the ground, I clamp his narrow waist between my thighs and squeeze until he shrieks. I love knowing I could snap his spine like a potato chip, and then, when he starts to cry, I love letting him go. We jump to our feet, and our eyes lock, dazzled, before I take off running, slaloming parked cars, his pack of friends just a clenched fist behind as I bolt across the street. We tear though backyard gardens, hurtle sandboxes, dodge swing sets until, one by one, the boys drop out of the chase, curses fizzling like damp fireworks in the sweetness of dusk.

I love the carefully printed notes he sends me afterward, signed with X's and O's, and the twin silver bracelets he steals from his mother's jewelry box and presents to me, wrapped in toilet paper and Scotch tape. He asks me if I'll go with him to Fish Day, Port Washington's annual summer festival. This is early June, and Fish Day isn't until late July, but that doesn't matter. My first date! And yet, I'm relieved when my mother says no, I'm too young to have a sweetheart. "Just tell him that July is a long time away," she suggests, but what I tell him is something I've read in a book: *Sorry, but your eyes are set too low for such a high fence.*

I love it that I'm not old enough for certain things, and that I'm still young enough for others, like taking my shirt off at Harrington Beach, where my girl-cousins and I, naked to the waist, splash through Lake Michigan's frigid shallows after schools of little fish. Now and then, we have to hop out and bury our aching feet in warm sand. I love that ache, how it feels worse before it feels better. I love the alewife stink of the beach, and its smooth, gray stones. High overhead, along the edge of the bluff, evergreens grow at terrible angles, like crooked teeth. Each spring, a few more come tumbling down, and another couple inches of Port Washington floats away.

I love the names of the little towns to the north: Dacada, Oostburg, Sheboygan. Sometimes, my brother and I ride our bikes to the farm in Knellsville where my father was born. We leave them hidden in a corn row while we enter the cool woods. Following deer paths, we make our way east until we reach the dropoff. Below is the shining platter of the lake. The shark fin of a sailboat. Further out, a barge with its dark load of coal. Our nostrils burn with the sharp, green sting of juniper bushes, and we rub the dusty berries between our fingers before scrabbling down the side of the bluff, clinging to exposed roots, grabbing branches, sliding the last ten feet on our butts. Already, we can hear the artesian well, buried somewhere deep in the haunch of the bluff. A stream of water runs clear and cold toward the lake, and we squat to drink from it, cupping our hands, pretending we are self-sufficient, survivors living off the land.

At night, my mother comes into our rooms to hear our bedtime prayers. When my father is home, he'll sometimes listen, too. But he stands in the doorway, shaking his head. He thinks my brother and I are too old for this.

"Are we too old?" I ask.

My mother says no. She explains that Grandpa and Grandma Ansay *never* tucked my father in, so he doesn't understand how important it is.

Sometimes, I feel very sorry for my father.

Dear God, I plead with the dark emptiness above my bed, *I'm sorry for all my sins. Please bless my mother and brother and father and me, and people here and on other planets, and all animals everywhere—*

I say the same thing every night, though "all animals everywhere" is a recent addition. Father Stone says that animals can't go to heaven, but I believe that if I pray, if I have faith, all things are possible.

—and please protect everybody who has died, and everybody who hasn't been born yet, and Satan—

After all, didn't God say to love all things? And wasn't

Satan one of his creatures? I have an idea that if everybody prays for him, Satan will come around to God's light once again, wake up as if splashed by cold water, and then there will be no more evil in the world. For a while, I'd been enlisting the help of kids at school, making them join hands to pray for Satan in the belly of the jungle gym, but then my teacher gave me a note, in a sealed envelope, to take home to my mother. So now, I pray for Satan in the privacy of my bedroom as my mother sits on the edge of my bed, listening calmly, rubbing my back. She has told me she prefers not to pray for Satan herself, but that I may do as I wish. When I'm finished, she kisses me, tucks the covers tight.

"Don't go yet," I say, but I know it's my brother's turn.

My mother winds the music box to conceal the sound of her footsteps moving away. Fear washes over me in shattering waves. I can't move. It's hard to breathe. Even before the music stops, my throat aches with unspeakable things.

Night after night, I struggle to fall asleep, to escape this paralyzing sense that something terrible is going to happen. And all it will take to stop it from happening is one small gesture on my part: holding my breath, or not holding my breath. Sleeping on my right side or sleeping on my left. Chanting eight Hail Marys, or four, or two—which is it? Sundays at Mass, I am so very careful to fold my hands with my right thumb crossed over my left, to let the Host dissolve in my mouth without brushing against my teeth, to genuflect all the way—knee touching ground—when I pass in front of the sanctuary.

Dear God, I pray, clutching my Saint Benedict medal, my rosary, the blessed icons glued to felt that Grandma Krier gives me for being a good girl. But I hear nothing but the drumming of my heartbeat, echoing deep within the coils of my mattress. And what if the sound isn't coming from my heart, but from Satan, who doesn't want to be saved, who is hiding there, waiting to get me, waiting to pull me down? Occasionally, this panic hits as I'm walking home from school, forcing me to count sidewalk cracks, the trees I pass, the number of steps I take. Even numbers are good, particularly fours and eights and twos; odd numbers are bad, particularly threes and sevens. If somebody gives me three cookies, I have to give one back. If my mother gives me a handful of chocolate chips, and I count twenty-seven, I must ask her to give me one more.

Why?

"Because something bad will happen if you don't," I explain.

My mother's face—I can see it now. Could it be she understands? She doesn't attempt to convince me otherwise. She gives me the extra chocolate chip.

As a child, I love my mother above all else, even my own self. Once, after reading the story of Isaac in the Bible—whose father, Abraham, is prepared, at God's request, to slaughter his bleating son like a goat—I asked her who she'd choose if she had to choose between God and me.

"God," she said, without looking at me, which was how I knew she meant it. "Because God came first. Without Him, neither of us would exist."

I nodded, pretending I understood, but a window of loneliness and sorrow opened up within me, opened and opened again until it consumed me from the inside out, and I stumbled away from her as if I'd caught fire: brilliant, blinding, inconsolable.

Four

GRANDMA KRIER SUBSCRIBED to a number of religious magazines and bulletins. She kept years' worth of back issues piled up in the utility bathroom, where we left our muddy boots before coming into the house. The cat box was there, too, along with sacks of litter and kibble, chicken feed from the mill, and, if there were new kittens, they slept with their mama on a blanket in the shower stall. People rarely used this bathroom, preferring the tidier one inside the main part of the house.

When I was in grade school, I spent many rainy afternoons curled up with or without kittens on the floor of the shower, reading through mildewy stacks of the *Catholic Digest.* Every issue was packed with miraculous falls and dramatic cures, illustrated with brightly colored disaster scenes. Skiers clung to broken ski lifts. Helicopters spiraled to the ground. An IV hung above a hospital bed, its occupant wrapped like a mummy.

Dear Jesus, What Should We Try Next? the captions read. *Lord, Help My Baby. There Was Nothing We Could Do For Mom But Pray.*

As I got older, it occurred to me that each of these stories was really the same one. The reading I'd done in grade school had prepared me to accept this, yet I couldn't help wondering if there wasn't something better out there. I'd long ago exhausted the children's corner at our local library; by the time I'd finished fifth grade, I'd read anything worth reading on the Young Adult shelf as well. Yet the main fiction section of the library overwhelmed me—how did I go about choosing one or two books out of so many? The summer before I started junior high, I came up with a system: I'd wander the aisles until I found a row of books that had all been written by the same author. My theory was that anyone who had published that much *had* to be good. I'd pull one at random and take it home.

But these books, too, were disappointing, though their covers alluded to an excitement earthier than anything the

Catholic Digest ever promised. Well-muscled men in torn shirts clutched beautiful, swooning women in their arms. A knife or a gun was usually close by; horses sometimes figured into things as well. Many of these novels seemed to take place during the Revolutionary War, though others featured rebellious slaves, settlers confronted by ketchup-colored Indians. A few were set in medieval times. Now and then, a vampire or a dragon cropped up, which required a stabbing or slaying. Ho hum. I found myself skipping pages, skimming for words like *bosom* or *loins:* the sex scenes, if not original, could often be instructive, although they had a way of dissolving into abstracts just at the point where my curiosity peaked.

Desperate, I turned to the books tucked away in my mother's hope chest. The hope chest was the only thing in the house, perhaps the only thing in my mother's entire life, which she'd asked my brother and me not to touch, using adult words like *privacy* and *respect,* so we'd understand how important this was to her. We promised and then, of course, we riffled through it as soon as we got the chance, indignant at the thought that she might try to keep secrets from us. The chest, I realize now, contained little; the bittersweet truth was that my mother had nothing to hide. Still, we rolled our eyes at the poetry she'd written to my father during their courtship, fingered the baby clothes she'd sewn for us, stared at the photographs of her father, our dead grandfather. We giggled over a little songbook in which my Uncle Don had printed neatly: *Sylvia is a fly.* Beneath it were a few musty-smelling paperbacks from her college English classes. These we'd passed back and forth uneasily, if they were pornography.

I choked on *Daisy Miller* but relished *Wuthering Heights, Jane Eyre,* and, especially, *An American Tragedy.* I lingered over the word *disrobe,* which I'd had to look up in the dictionary, and then I read the scene again and again. How was it, I wondered, that a single word could be more titillating than strings of adverbs? How could I dislike Clyde Griffiths so and, yet, feel sorry for him too? How was it I could finish a book's final chapter and find myself left with more questions than I'd had at the beginning? Difficult questions, too. I sucked each one like an unfamiliar brand of hard candy, not certain if I liked the flavor, yet unable to spit it out. The characters stayed with me in a ghostly kind of way, especially those I hadn't agreed with, hadn't fully understood. I found myself thinking about them off and on throughout the day, the way I thought about people I actually knew. And yet, I wasn't sure how reading about such people, *real* people, made me feel. I wasn't sure if it wasn't, just maybe, a slightly immoral thing to do.

Until now, everything I'd ever read—from the Bible to books assigned in school—had reinforced what I'd been taught to believe: good people get rewarded; bad people get punished. Once you knew who was who, you could stop reading if you wanted. You could figure out, from that point on, how the book was going to end. Even my well-thumbed copy of the *Lives of the Saints* had started to leave me cold. Despite the wonderfully gruesome tortures, you knew from the start that Faith would triumph, so what was the point of reading further?

No one had ever actively discouraged me from reading. No one had ever actively discouraged me from drinking coffee, either. A cup now and then, with plenty of milk and sugar, was absolutely fine for a child. Too much, however, risked stunted growth or discolored teeth. Too many books risked *bookishness,* which led to *acting too big for your britches* or, worse, *putting on airs*—a tendency toward which I already leaned. And, too, reading the wrong book—like visiting somebody else's church—could lead to confusion that over time might crack the foundation of even the soundest faith.

If my mother noticed me reading on the couch, that was fine, but if I was still there an hour later, mouth open, immune to the world, she was quick to find something else for me to do. Something that involved, say, a pair of my father's old BVDs soaked in lemon Pledge, or the vacuum cleaner. Nothing irked her more than the sight of me lying around the house with a book, except, perhaps, when she caught me and my brother watching "the boob tube" without permission. Our house was in a neighborhood teeming with other kids: Why not go outside and play? What about a game of tennis at the junior high athletic field across the street? Weed the garden. Fill the bird feeder. Or, shovel the sidewalk. For Pete's sake, *do* something.

Even I could see that reading was a kind of mental nap, the sort of activity the Bible called *sloth,* a habit that led nowhere. At the time, I was planning to become a heart surgeon, much to my father's delight. It was his suggestion that I look for books about medicine, doctors, sickness. This was an idea my mother liked, too. Ask the librarian to recommend something, she said.

The librarian did.

For the rest of the summer, I read books about crippled children with heroic personalities. The particulars of each story varied, but the general plot was always the same. A child with a birth defect is born into an unsuspecting family. (Variation: an innocent child suffers an injury, or develops a rare disease.) At first, the family is left reeling from the blow. Relatives and well-meaning friends suggest that the child be institutionalized. Doctors throw up their hands and walk away. But, thanks to the power of faith (variation: positive thinking and perseverance), the family rallies around the child, discovering in the process that instead of a tragedy, this child is the greatest blessing of their lives. Shortly thereafter, a miracle occurs. The child who would never be able to walk, walks. The mute girl speaks. The boy who the very best specialists insist will never recognize his mother, looks up at her one day and smiles.

Again, I skimmed, this time in search of medical details. I learned about cerebral palsy, spina bifida, muscular dystrophy, cystic fibrosis, leukemia. I liked to imagine myself stricken with one of those diseases: how brave and cheerful I'd be! Of course, I'd offer up all my sufferings to the Poor Souls in Purgatory, and when I died, these liberated souls—I imagined them as flat, white disks, sort of like fancy dinner plates—would meet me at heaven's gate. God, moved by this display, would ask me if I needed anything from earth to be more comfortable with Him in the afterlife, and I'd eloquently make a case for admitting animals. These daydreams were far more satisfying than the stories that had inspired them, and I was happy enough to return the books when school started again in the fall. There, in sixth-grade English, our first reading assignment was Ray Bradbury's "The Veldt." I liked the story well enough, but I'd read it the year before. Already, I knew by heart everything I was supposed to write about it, everything the teacher wanted me to say.

* * *

A month or so after school had started, I was walking home one day when a rummage sale caught my eye. I loved rummage sales. I loved walking up a stranger's driveway, looking in the garage, snooping around their stuff. I loved pawing through the mismatched china, chipped figurines, and vacation souvenirs. Usually, I glanced through the water-stained paperbacks, historical novels, romances, all the covers I recognized. But today, I saw a different sort of book, a fat hardback with a glossy jacket. It was called *The Chosen*. Something about its cover brought to mind the books in my mother's hope chest.

I picked it up.

I almost put it down because I couldn't pronounce the author's name—*Chaim Potok?* (I sounded it out: *Chame Poh-tick?*) But the plot had to do with a friendship between two Jewish boys, and now I knew I would *have* to read this book because I'd just met a Jewish a girl named Roberta, who had been my desk partner at the beginning of the year. I had liked Roberta because she played the violin, and because she wasn't embarrassed to admit she was good at it. We'd even made plans to learn Kreisler's Praeludium and Allegro together. But she and her family had stayed in Port for only a month before putting their house back on the market and returning to Milwaukee, where they'd come from. It was just "too difficult," Roberta had said, and I'd nodded as if I understood. The truth was that before I'd met Roberta, I'd always thought of Jews as Bible story people, like David and Goliath, or Jonah and the whale—people who, like angels, had lived long ago. Every year at Easter time, there was a moment of silence during Mass in which we "prayed for the Jews, who were the chosen people." As I prayed, I'd imagine people wrapped in flowing white bed sheets, wearing sandals and halos made from pipe cleaners and glitter—the costumes we kids wore on All Saints' Day when we paraded into the church to the hymn "When the Saints Come Marching In."

The chosen people. *The Chosen.* Though I didn't know the word *allusion,* I recognized the concept with a little thrill of pleasure. I dug a quarter out of the pocket of my jeans, paid for the book, and started reading as I walked home.

Nothing in my life thus far could have prepared me for the world I was about to enter. *The Chosen* begins with a baseball game in the Williamsburg section of Brooklyn, shortly after America's entry into World War II. Danny, the oldest son of a Hasidic rabbi, is batting for the Hasidic yeshiva's team; Reuven is pitching for a progressive Orthodox yeshiva. Early in the game, things turn ugly, and when Danny hits the ball directly at Reuven, Reuven refuses to duck. The ball shatters his glasses, and he is nearly blinded as a result. Danny visits Reuven at the hospital, and the two boys become friends. It's a friendship that revolves around learning, around books, around intellectual challenges, and I quickly realized that the verb *study,* in this world, didn't mean simply opening some books for an hour or two after supper. Danny and Reuven *devour* books, discuss them, argue about them, even as they reach for more. And their families seem to think that this is all perfectly normal. In fact, kids are expected to spend practically every waking hour analyzing religious texts and pondering heady mathematics. But when Danny starts to study psychology, he must keep this a secret from his religious father, for it is Danny's birthright, as the oldest son, to become a rabbi. Soon it becomes clear that the ideas he's encountering—those of Freud among them—can only lead him away from his faith.

Now here was something I recognized, a fear I'd been raised with, one that occupied a powerful cornerstone of my consciousness. To *lose your faith* was worse, I believed, than anything, even death. Why would Danny risk it? I read and reread all the scenes in which he and Reuven study together. I tasted the sweet, unfamiliar diction of their daily lives: *tzaddik, gematriya, apikorsim, tzitzit.* I lingered just as ardently over the names of great philosophers—*Kant, Spinoza, Aristotle,* names that I'd never heard before, names that the context of the prose made clear were not by any means obscure. Too much, too much, I could not absorb it all, and yet I couldn't stop reading, couldn't make myself stop to breathe, digest. I noticed that there were quite a few political arguments between various characters, and that these arguments were sprinkled with words like *Zion* and *Israel*—words I recognized from the Bible—but I couldn't figure out what they meant in this context, or what, exactly, was at stake. I recognized the name of President Roosevelt. I recognized the name of Hitler. Neither of these names meant anything significant to me. Roosevelt had led the United States; Hitler had led Germany. But who, exactly, were the Allies? The United Nations? What was a "European Jewry"? It was all very confusing, and whenever I hit a long passage about the war, I skipped it, eager to get back to Reuven and Danny, their personal stories, their studies, their friendship.

How can it be that, at the age of eleven—a sixth-grade student—I knew so little of history, even less of politics, nothing at all about the Nazis? In our small, predominantly German community, there'd been little discussion of *either* world war. We studied Alexander the Great. We studied the Ottoman Empire. At one point, I remember memorizing a long poem that began "I hope the old Romans had painful ab-domens; I hope that the Greeks had toothaches for weeks; I hope the Egyptians had chronic conniptions; I hope that the Vandals had thorns in their sandals . . ." But what I remember best is how we studied the Civil War. We couldn't get enough of hearing about it. It was better than a bedtime story. We, the virtuous North, had fought the evil South—and won! And we'd done so simply out of the goodness of our hearts, to free the helpless Negroes.

At one point, a guidance counselor came to our classroom, and we played a special game in which half the class got a blue pin to wear and the other half got a red pin. The people with the red pins had to do whatever the blue pins said. Then the guidance counselor said, "Switch!" and the blue pins got to boss the red pins around. We loved it! We begged to do it again!

"Now you know what it was like to be a slave," the guidance counselor said. "It's hard to understand, in this day and age, how anyone could treat another human being that way."

***The Chosen* stayed** with me like a country I had visited, a place I'd stayed just long enough to be disoriented, shocked, by what I saw upon my return home. I thought about Danny and Reuven when my history teacher raised the map at the front of the classroom, and burst into tears at the sight of a grotesque vulva chalked on the blackboard beneath. I thought about it in the art room when Lewis Dolittle sucked a mouthful of water from the spigot, and spat it in the face of a particularly quiet girl for no reason other than meanness. I thought about it in math class, where we were reviewing long division yet again; I thought about it when our principal called me out of class to reprimand me for requesting permission to take a foreign language class with the eight graders. Awfully big for my britches, wasn't I? Well, he wasn't about to put up with this nonsense! No ma'am, I could take a foreign language when I got to eighth grade like the rest of my classmates. Who did I think I was, acting as if I were better than everyone else?

I thought about *The Chosen* walking home after school, leaving by the side door to avoid the popular kids, cutting through the clouds of cigarette and pot smoke released by the stoners. I even thought about it at the piano where, usually, nothing could distract me. I understood, for the first time, what literature could be: an opportunity to live beyond yourself, to be bigger and brighter than you'd ever hoped to be. To see your face reflected back, framed within a broader context. To stare at that reflection, and begin to dream.

"Is everything all right at school?" my mother said.

"Everything's fine," I said.

* * *

I decided that I would teach myself to study the way Reuven and Danny studied. I would make study part of my daily life, like prayer, like practicing the piano.

I had a desk in my bedroom. It was white, with baby blue drawers and gilded drawer pulls. It didn't seem like the kind of desk Reuven and his father would have used, but I figured it would have to do. First thing Saturday morning, I cleaned out the drawers, wiped the top with Windex. I set out a single, pristine notebook, a couple of freshly sharpened pencils, and my copy of *The Chosen.* Then I set about hunting down the dictionary. I discovered it with the Scrabble board, in the cupboard underneath the wet bar, where we kept the rest of the household's intellectual property: the Bible, the *World Book Encyclopedia,* a guide to seashell identification, and my father's plastic label-maker. The dictionary's cover was missing, and the front pages were lined with Scrabble scores, but its insides were intact.

When I had my desk set up, I paged through *The Chosen* and made a list of the scholars and philosophers Danny and Reuven had mentioned. Then I stuck the list in my pocket, put on my coat, and headed for the library. I hadn't bothered writing down the names of any fiction writers; I was done with such frivolous study. I was going to dedicate myself to psychology, religion, and mathematics. But when I opened the card catalogue, I discovered there were no books by Freud in our library. There were no books by Aristotle, or Spinoza, or Kant; there was no copy of *Principia Mathematica.* Reuven had been reading a book on logic by Susanne Langer: no listing. Danny had been upset by a writer named Graetz: nothing. It crossed my mind that I could simply study the Talmud. But when I asked at the desk, the librarian, without changing expression, said that she'd never heard of such a book. Who'd written it again? she said, and I said I wasn't sure, but I thought it was like the Bible, that nobody had written it.

God, the librarian informed me, had written the Bible.

I wandered back to the card catalogue. Briefly, I considered reading the Bible, but it seemed too ordinary, too familiar; I wanted to start with something that would shake me up, the way Freud had shaken up Danny. It occurred to me that Chaim Potok might have invented the books he'd mentioned in *The Chosen,* the way he'd invented Danny and Reuven. But no—I knew that Freud, at least, was real. He was the guy who'd figured out that what girls really wanted were penises. Even I knew that. It didn't seem to me that *I'd* ever wanted a penis, though I could clearly remember a group of us girls teasing Buddy Burmiester because we could have babies and he couldn't. This had been in fourth grade. We'd taunted him until he cried. But maybe things had been different in Freud's day.

Not that I was going to be able to read him and find out for myself.

I thought as hard as I could, riffling through the flotsam and jetsam of six years of public school education. Somewhere in all that, there had to be another name I might look up, someone whose writings I might study. I looked up Alexander Graham Bell. I looked up George Washington and Abraham Lincoln. There was a book *about* Benjamin Franklin, but that had been checked out. *Think,* I told myself sternly. And then I came up with another name, one that had even been mentioned in *The Chosen.*

Adolf Hitler.

Why *was* that name so familiar? I had a vague grade school memory of a group of boys marching around on the playground, kicking their legs and shouting *Heil Hitler!* until the teachers made them stop. The name triggered a sense of power and importance. I knew that Hitler was a German, like Freud, like me—my father's maternal grandparents and my mother's paternal grandparents had been born in Germany—and like almost everybody in our small community. I knew from reading *The Chosen* that he'd been on the losing side of World War II, a war that, according to one of my aunts, had been "greatly exaggerated." She'd said this at my grandmother's house, in front of a number of my aunts and uncles, and I could tell from the beat of silence that followed that she'd said something inappropriate, something—maybe rude? I couldn't tell. At any rate, it was clear that nobody wanted to talk about it. Everybody smiled until the conversation turned to something else.

I pulled out the H drawer, flicked through the cards. I was in luck. Adolf Hitler had written one book, *Mein Kampf*, translated into English as *My Struggle*. Our library had a copy.

The expressionless librarian checked me out.

I began the book as soon as I got home, looking up words I didn't know and copying definitions into my notebook. It was rather dry going, but I kept at it, and I didn't let myself skip ahead, for I knew from reading *The Chosen* that there were times when Reuven, and even brilliant Danny, had spent entire days on one paragraph. I believe there was an introduction of some kind, and in my mind's eye, there are reproductions of a few of Hitler's landscape paintings—but I may have superimposed some later memory, something I saw in a college course, over this earlier one. I do believe I learned a few things about art. I learned about the death of Hitler's mother. I sensed that neither topic was the point of the book, but I couldn't tell what was coming, where all the rambling observations were leading. It was certainly different from the novels I'd read.

At last, I stopped reading and went over my list of vocabulary words: one, I think, was *oratory.* Then I planned out my assignment for the next day.

I had studied for one hour—an hour I usually spent at the piano.

I had hoped that, during the night, things I hadn't understood about the book would come clear. Instead, I found my second session even more challenging than the first. I began to flip ahead, I couldn't help myself, and encountered a brief scene in which Hitler is walking down the street and sees a Jewish man walking toward him. Just like that, he knows the man is "vermin." I looked up "vermin," copied down its definitions: noxious or objectionable animals or insects, including rats and worms and parasites; objectionable, filthy persons.

Hmm, I thought. The man must have done something to make Hitler angry. But, studying the little scene again, I found nothing in the text but a description of the man's face.

A strange, uneasy feeling swept over me. I pushed it away. Surely, I must have missed something. Surely there must be some rational explanation for what Hitler believed. That was why it was important not to skip ahead. I sighed. There was nothing to do but reread the book from the beginning and catch whatever it was. So I began again. It was a Sunday afternoon; the house was still. My brother was down in his basement room. My father had gone to the office. My mother was taking a nap. Sounds seemed louder than usual: the hum of the refrigerator in the kitchen, the thrum of the heat kicking in, the click in my throat whenever I swallowed.

What had the Jewish man done? Why couldn't I see it?

Again, I began to skip ahead, unable to follow the sentences. Again, I came to the section in which the word "vermin" appeared. Hitler, I thought. Adolf Hitler. I thought about the boys on the playground, the expressions on the teachers' faces when they'd made them stop chanting and shouting. An expression that was guarded and thin-lipped and close. The expression they got whenever somebody used a bad word, or if somebody asked a question that nobody wanted to answer. The expression I'd seen at my grandmother's house on the day that my aunt had said World War II was "greatly exaggerated."

I reached for my copy of *The Chosen* and began flipping through it, skimming for the word "Hitler," searching out the very pages I'd skipped—pages that had to do with the war. *Six million Jews slaughtered,* I found. *Gas chambers. Hitler's ovens.* The words sounded cartoonish, like something Wile E. Coyote might think up. Like something out of a nightmare. Like something a crazy person might do.

Fear seized the back of my neck as if it were a black-gloved hand. I jumped up and sat down and jumped up again. Then I shoved *My Struggle* into the bottom of my backpack. I carried it out of my room, down the stairs and through the foyer, where I shoved it to the back of the coat closet with the stack of newspapers for recycling.

The next day, after school, I took it back to the library. I threw out the notebook with the vocabulary words; I put the dictionary back in the cupboard. That was the year I increased my piano practice from one to two hours each day. That was the year I decided I didn't want to be a heart surgeon anymore. I certainly didn't want to be a scholar or philosopher. I stopped going to the library. I didn't read another book, beyond what a teacher assigned, for the next ten years.

Vermin: even now, that word holds it power, moves from my mouth like some living, whiskered thing that brushed against me in the dark.

Part Two

Five

People looked at me strangely when I said loved to practice the piano. Were my parents pushing me to do it? Wasn't it hard to rush home from school, day after day, instead of spending time with friends? Two hours a day, three hours a day. I'd sit down at the keyboard, and blink, and somehow the time had passed. I loved to practice in the same way that someday, as an adult, I would love to write. Only then it would be publication that left me uneasy. As a child, it was performing I disliked.

I'd stand there, in the wings, in the deep black box of all that might happen, all that could go wrong. The curtains swayed slightly, humming with the sound of the audience, a sound that is strangely like a rookery, a flock of birds arranging themselves for the night. Sometimes, though I wasn't supposed to, I'd peer out from the edge of the stage and there they'd be: strangers stepping over each other's knees, unbuttoning coats, opening programs. When I stepped back into the darkness, I'd see purple and yellow rings. And then, gradually, the piano, lit like an altar at the center of the stage.

If there was time, I'd duck out to the rest room and soak my hands in hot water. Bending over the basin, I stared at myself in the mirror: beetle-browed, long-jawed, absolutely serious. Cropped fingernails. Gold cross at my throat. I was twelve, I was fourteen, I was sixteen. *Dear God,* I'd pray, *help me to stay focused, help me to concentrate, help me*—yes, I prayed this as well—*to be a better person.* It all seemed connected somehow. If I was good, if I was worthy, I'd perform well—how could I not? I prayed until the water in the basin cooled and I felt the familiar lightness enter my bones, illuminating me with such weight, such absolute purpose and calm, that I could see the notes spread out before me as clearly as I saw the wrinkles in my fingertips. I believed that this feeling was Grace. I believed that it came from God, the way I believed that all good things came from God, the way I believed that all bad things came from within myself, my flawed human frailty. If anyone had suggested to me, then, that I was summoning my own strength, my own capabilities, I would have been horrified.

Somewhere between sixth and eighth grade, I had fundamentally changed. At school, I'd stopped arguing with my teachers; I no longer bothered to raise my hand. At home, I shrugged, said little, kept my opinions to myself. I was weak, I was nothing—or at least, that's what I was trying to be. And whenever I failed, asserted myself, began a sentence with the words *I want,* a voice in my head was certain to chide me: *Watch out what you want, or you'll get it.* It was arrogant to want, to expect, to choose. Only God, all-knowing and omnipotent, could know what was best for anybody. I put myself in His hands. I turned myself over to God.

The moment any child, male or female, first learns to envision God as male, some crucial part of his or her imagination is forever damaged, limited, changed. The moment a female child credits a male god for all that is beautiful and good while simultaneously accepting responsibility for all that is sinful—literally, all that "misses the mark"—she has internalized a particularly dangerous self-loathing. As a little girl, I'd wanted to be the fastest, the smartest, the strongest; now, instead of leaping forward, I held back, prayed for guidance, and whenever I listened for an answer, it was a masculine voice I longed to hear. As my body matured, and I began to think of myself less as a "kid" and more as a "girl," I felt myself to be growing apart from God, more differentiated from His image. If God was perfection, then my adolescent female body was an exaggeration of *im*perfection. The only course of action was to abandon myself whenever possible, to become *by choice* an empty vessel, like the Virgin Mary, for whom I was named, and upon whom I—like so many Catholic girls—was encouraged to model myself.

A virgin *and* a mother as a teenage role model?

For those who do believe, no explanation is necessary, I was told. *For those who don't believe, no explanation is possible.*

Throughout my adolescence, I lived in two worlds that could not be reconciled: the world as it was presented to me, a world I was told to accept on faith, and a second world, the world of my reasoning, the world of empirical experience. I did the best I could to shut out the second world, to be a good daughter, a good Catholic, to become that empty vessel for Our Lord. Yet what to do with everything I felt: passion and violence, wonder and despair? Music was a means of being simultaneously empty and full-to-bursting. Music gave voice to everything I wasn't permitted to feel and think and say. When I finished playing, I'd simply close the lid and walk away. I considered myself His instrument. I claimed none of that joyful noise as my own.

I dried my hands, stretched my fingers, rubbed my tender forearms. Warm-ups, my teachers said, prevented tendinitis, but it didn't seem to matter if I warmed up or not. If I spent the weekend at my grandmother's farm, where there was no piano, the tenderness went away. But it always came right back as soon as I started to practice again. I was proud of my pain, my ability to take it. I thought it was romantic. It was only natural that God would ask you to suffer for something you loved. Jesus, after all, had loved Mary above all other women, and Jesus had allowed Mary to suffer more than anyone—as a sign of His favor, Father Stone explained. It was Saturday catechism. It was nothing we hadn't heard before in that overheated basement room. We stared dully at Father, lined up in our rows, puddles shining around our boots. He smiled at us encouragingly, as if there were no contradiction in what he'd just said, as if it made perfect sense. "Does anyone have any questions?" he'd always ask at the end of each session, but none of us ever did.

Love was pain. Suffering without resistance was proof of devotion to God. You did not think about the way such beliefs would undercut your ability to protect yourself, assert yourself, excel. The meek, after all, would inherit the earth. The saints wore their mortifications like jewels about their murdered necks.

Sometimes there'd be an introduction before the performance, sometimes not. Sometimes I'd be one of several performers, one of many performers, one of any number of variety acts that could range from religious recitations to a duet played on kazoos. Sometimes I'd perform at luncheons, at schools and colleges, at fund-raisers and churches. Sometimes I'd play in master classes, in which case the audience would consist of other musicians, all of them older than I was. Afterward, there'd be questions for the teacher, and I'd be asked to repeat certain passages so the teacher could reiterate my weaknesses, assign technical exercises, suggest particular additions to my repertoire.

Sometimes I'd play in competitions, and sometimes these competitions were "blind," meaning that the judge or judges were not supposed to know who was playing, and so they'd be seated behind a screen. But if you looked, afterward, you'd see them peeking, see in their faces where you stood. Sometimes the pianos were exactly what you'd expect: a beat-up Kawai at the back of a school cafeteria; a buttery Steinway L in the lakefront home where I entertained a private party at Christmastime. And sometimes, the pianos caught you off guard: at the Milwaukee cathedral, another Steinway, this time with the brassy intonation of a jackhammer. At a run-down recording studio, a honey-colored Schimmel with an exquisite, piercing treble—even now, eighteen years later, I can reproduce that tone in my mind. A sturdy little Yamaha in an airport hotel where, at seventeen, I would run through my college audition pieces one last time.

Each piano is unique. Each feels different beneath your hand and yields a new geography of sound. Each room or hall accepts that sound in a completely different way, and if, within that room or hall, the piano is moved, the sound will change, as it will if the hall is full of people in thick winter coats, or half full of people in light summer dresses. You must adjust your touch, your tone, your range; you must *listen,* for even the most familiar passages can become unfamiliar, challenging, strange. Performing on an unknown piano means making these adjustments instantly, fluidly, anticipating how to handle the upcoming measures based on the few you've just played. A light touch that on my home piano created a nimble pianissimo could result, on stage, in galumphing gap-toothed runs, the fourth fingers slurring notes, the weighty thumbs oversounding. What were full, ringing chords in my teacher's studio might become, in regional competition, a battery of gunshot slaps.

"You were *banging,*" my teachers would tell me afterward, or else, "What happened to your *singing legato?*" Perhaps my *staccato* was *lazy.* Perhaps I got too excited and my *mezzoforte* came out *forte* or, worse, *fortissimo,* and I still had a true *fortissimo* coming up—but I hadn't been able to deliver.

"You *held nothing back,*" my teachers would scold. "You *left yourself nowhere to go.*"

I was twenty-five when I first encountered a one-page story by Kafka in which a cat chases a mouse down a long hall. The walls are narrowing, narrowing—the walls of any nightmare—until at last they meet and the mouse is trapped.

"It's not fair!" the mouse cries. "There was nowhere else to go!"

"All you had to do was change directions," the cat says.

And then he eats the mouse.

It is always a question of imagination, of knowing which direction to turn, how to interpret what you see.

I taped a postcard of Carnegie Hall to the white, quilted headboard over my bed, just beneath the prayer card Grandma Krier had given me, printed with the twenty-first Psalm. On my nightstand, next to a porcelain figurine of Mary holding Baby Jesus, I kept a hollow bank in the shape of a Tootsie Pop, stuffed with my baby-sitting money, and labeled JUILLIARD FUND. I practiced finger exercises on my desk at school, got permission to carry my sack lunch to the music room, where I disrupted the harassed choir director's only peaceful hour. When I practiced well, I felt light and sober, clean. The very air seemed to shine. When I played badly, I felt as if I were moving underwater, weighed down, distorted by all the things I could not say, questions I was not supposed to ask. Because one question led to another, and suddenly the entire fabric of your faith, your life, began to unravel before your eyes.

Away from the piano, I moved like a sleepwalker through the honey-brown molasses of each day: prayers before and after meals, prayers again at bedtime, Wednesday night devotions, Sunday morning Mass. The clock in the steeple of Saint Mary's Church stared down on us all, merciless and unblinking, from its perch overlooking the town. In January, spit froze when it hit the sidewalk; in July, the air was hot, damp, still. Schools of alewives washed up on the beach, the stench like a shimmering cloud, buoyed by the roar of flies. Nights, when lightning carved up the sky, we hurried down to the basement with blankets and a crackling transistor radio. Too soon, summer passed back into autumn, that brief, brilliant fire; I dozed through the long, empty hours of school. By the end of October, there were snow flurries, and soon the white walls of winter descended: smothering as God's will. The lake froze. Fishermen dragged out their shanties. On New Year's Day, people drove their cars out on the ice. There were two grocery stores in our town, a bowling alley, a row of struggling shops on Main. There were seven churches. There were nearly a dozen bars, but I wasn't old enough to drink.

At the end of each summer, my mother drove my brother and me to Milwaukee to shop for school clothes. She made us sit in the backseat and put our seatbelts on. As soon as she'd entered the city limits, she turned off the radio and forbade us to speak, hugging the right lane so she wouldn't have to pass. Her foot rode the brake. When we got to the mall, she circled the parking lot until she found a space beneath a light. Inevitably, we all had to run back to double-check that the doors and windows were locked.

We rarely left the Port Washington area. "If Port don't got it, you don't need it," people said, and for our purposes, this was true. Even my piano lessons had always been in town. My teacher was the music director at our church; I came to her when I was six, studied with her until the summer before I started high school.

When I was three, when we'd still lived in Michigan, my mother had tried to enroll me with another piano teacher, but was told that a child too young to say her alphabet was far too young for the piano. In fact, I could say the alphabet, but one of this teacher's rules had been that parents could not be present during lessons—too distracting—and as soon as my mother left, I promptly forgot "Silent Night" and "O Come, O Come, Emmanuel" and the melodies I'd gleaned from a boxed set called *Beethoven's Best Piano Sonatas*.

Rainy afternoons, I'd slide the cool black records from their sleeves and listen to what I called *dizzy music*. My mother pulled the coffee table out of harm's way, shoved the couch back with a well-placed bump of her hip, and my brother and I would spin until we staggered and fell to the floor. There we continued spinning on our hands and knees, the tops of our heads pressed to the carpet so that when the record ended and we sat upright, our fine hair rose and crackled with static electricity. Hour after hour we listened and spun to the Moonlight Sonata, to the Pathétique, to the Appassionata, but mostly—especially—to the Waldstein. I remember how badly I wanted more dizzy music, how I begged for it. But at Christmastime, I received a copy of Burl Ives's "The Lollipop Tree" instead.

Bach, Mozart, Rachmaninoff—these names, though my mother had heard of them, must have seemed as unreachable, as unrelated to our lives as the names comprising the periodic table of the elements. She longed for culture in an abstract way, but it was a longing she could neither justify nor explain, and on those rare occasions she took a risk, attempted something new—bought a stylish coat, ordered a series of faux-leather-bound books on the Roman Empire, attempted a recipe from a magazine—her efforts were inevitably unsuccessful. They became the butt of family jokes. The coat's lining tore the first time she wore it. The books gathered dust on the shelf. My father came home to the stir-fry or curry—both radical departures from our standard meat and potatoes fare—and said the first thing that flew into his head: "Whew! What's that smell?"

Like Kafka's mouse, my mother didn't know what to imagine, so she kept on running in the only direction she could. But my piano teacher had seen something more of the world. She loaned me records. She took me to the Pabst Theatre in Milwaukee where, at nine, I heard my first concert. She organized public recitals, made each of her students practice walking across a stage without scurrying or slouching, taught us to bow gracefully, one cool hand on the back of our necks. She urged us to attend music camp at the University of Wisconsin–Steven's Point. I went for the first time when I was ten and, abruptly, college became a real place, a concrete pursuit, with solid walls, tables, and chairs, a bustling sense of purpose.

Each year, one or two children were chosen to give special recitals and receive master classes with the Japanese instructors. The summer I turned twelve, I was one of them. Speaking through a translator, the teacher had stressed to my mother and me the importance of exposure to concerts and recitals, opera and the ballet. We'd nodded as if such things were an option. Of course, we *could* have driven to Milwaukee, or even Chicago, but at the time such an idea—had it even occurred to us—would have been dismissed as outrageous, a sinful extravagance, evidence that we were putting ourselves above regular people.

I loved the years I studied with my first teacher. I loved her for her precision, her intensity, the way she always took me very seriously, but also for her playfulness, her passion for the absurd. Sometimes, without warning, she'd drop a handful of music on the floor, trying to break my concentration. She'd stamp her feet, laugh raucously, sing out, "Mommy, I have to go to the bathroom!" Playing the piano required "absolute attention," a phrase she would often repeat. Years later, I'd encounter that phrase again: the French philosopher Simone Weil's definition of prayer.

So it was with "absolute attention" that I worked my way through all the Suzuki books, the Chopin nocturnes, Bach preludes and fugues, sonatas by Mozart and Beethoven. I was thirteen when my teacher informed my mother that I needed more advanced instruction: I not only had a solid repertoire but I could withstand any distraction without missing a single note.

"You mean another teacher?" my mother said.

There was somebody in Skokie, Illinois, my teacher said. Just outside Chicago, about two hours away. Miss Williams had an excellent reputation; her students went on to attend the best conservatories. One had been a finalist for the Van Cliburn. She herself toured internationally with a chamber ensemble.

Chicago? my mother said.

I had been to Chicago once, on a field trip. My fifth-grade class had gone to the Museum of Science and Industry. We'd had to hold hands with our buddy the whole time, and stay with the group, and not speak to strangers, and sound off by twos whenever the teacher said.

Think about your future, my teacher told me. Think about what you want.

My mother and I walked home together. She'd been coming to lessons with me, taking notes so she could help me with my practicing. Lately it had seemed to me, to all of us, that I had stalled somehow. I could manage the notes, but the pieces were exceeding my emotional capabilities. My sight-reading skills were terribly poor; I still played almost everything by ear. And then, too, there was the question of my technique, which my teacher feared might be causing my forearms to ache the way they did. A more advanced teacher might be able to see what was triggering the problem.

I wanted to go to Chicago for lessons every bit as badly as I wanted my mother to say it was out of the question, too expensive, time consuming, extravagant—which I knew was the truth. My mother had summers off from teaching, but she was getting more involved in my father's real estate company. She designed, wrote, and coordinated the weekly advertisement. She composed and typed most of my father's correspondence. She'd just started studying for her broker's license, which she hoped to earn before it was time to return to her classroom in fall. And in fall I, too, was going to be busy. At least, I hoped that would be the case. Surely, there'd be more homework in high school, more responsibilities, more interesting extracurriculars, than there'd been in junior high.

Any of these were perfectly acceptable reasons not to go to Chicago. But I knew there was another, more pressing reason.

My mother was afraid to drive me there.

"What do you want to do?" she said as we turned into the driveway.

"I don't know," I said.

"You'll have to do better than that," she said.

We were each waiting, as we often did, for the other to say what *she* wanted.

"We could try it for a while," I said.

Over dinner, during a commercial break, my mother told my father about Miss Williams, repeating the things that my teacher had told us. That if I wanted a career in music, it was important to make these decisions now. That Miss Williams had placed students at conservatories like Peabody, Curtis, even The Juilliard. That I'd have chances to compete, to perform, that a local teacher could not give me. Even if I eventually decided against a career in music, my mother said, such experiences would be invaluable—didn't my father agree? They could lead to other opportunities. They would affect me for the rest of my life.

My father said nothing. His eyes were on the TV. I remember that one of the commercials was for shampoo. I remember what we were eating that night: meat loaf, made with ground beef, stale bread, ketchup, egg, a packet of Lipton's onion soup. I felt like a character in a play, as if all of us were larger than life, significant, observed, and this self-consciousness embarrassed me. I tried to pray: *Dear God, make him say yes.* But that felt even more ridiculous. It was crazy to drive more than two hours each way for lessons that probably cost—what? My teacher charged seven dollars for an hour lesson that usually ran an hour and a half. I had, I realized, only been thinking of the cost in terms of time and gasoline.

"Skokie, Illinois," my father finally said. He stabbed at his baked potato a few times. "I know Skokie very well."

The news came back on.

This was a typical conversation with my father.

After supper, I cleared my father and brother's plates along with my own, clattering them around more than necessary as I rinsed them and put them in the dishwasher. My mother, who'd started the pots and pans, tried to catch my eye, but I kept my head down. I was furious: with myself, with my mother, and, especially, with my teacher. The whole idea was stupid. There had been no point in bringing it up in the first place.

And yet, I wanted my father to *acknowledge* that we had spoken to him. I wanted him to address the question my mother had asked on my behalf, even though I knew his mind simply did not work that way. I knew because I was wired the same way. If something caught my attention, I could concentrate on it for hours, to the exclusion of everything and everyone else, and still emerge burning, hungry for more, irritable at the interruption. But if I wasn't particularly interested, or if I happened to be thinking of something else, I found it nearly impossible to focus, to narrow all the possibilities into a single, specific answer.

We always ate promptly at five-thirty. Tonight, we had the dishes finished by six.

"I'm going to practice," I said.

But within minutes of completing my warm-ups, I broke a piano key. It was near the center of the keyboard, which meant that I wouldn't be able to practice again until the piano tuner had come. This could take up to a week. The piano was the same obliging little upright that my mother had learned to play on as a child, but lately it had been suffering under my relentless attacks. I stared at the deflated key as if I could heal it by the force of my will. I wished I knew somebody else who had a piano. I wished I could go out to the garage and get the heavy maul and break my mother's sweet piano into a thousand pieces.

When I looked up, I saw that my father was watching me. He had his shoes on and he held a clipboard in his hand.

"We need to call the tuner," I said. But my father didn't seem to notice.

"Let's go for a ride," he said.

When my father asked you to go for a ride, what he meant was that he wanted you to come with him on a property appraisal. I liked going on appraisals, walking through unfamiliar houses, holding the end of the tape measure. I liked hearing my father's assessment of each house: learning what was a selling point, what might be a drawback. But I hated getting in a car without knowing where, exactly, I would be going, and how long I was going to be. Forcing my father to answer either of these questions in advance was nearly impossible.

"What's the address?" I said, buckling my seatbelt. My father never wore his.

"The address," my father repeated. He backed out of the driveway and we headed north, through town. It was a warm summer evening, and everybody was out, families riding their bicycles, children playing in the streets. My father drove slowly, waving like the president. He knew nearly everyone in town.

"Is it far?" I said.

"Oh," he said. "Not far."

He pulled over to talk to a man who was thinking of putting his house on the market. He cut through a side street to check on one of his rental properties. "Tenant's home," he said, with satisfaction. "They're good people. If I could find half a dozen just like 'em . . ." He didn't finish what he was saying, for he'd been distracted by a woman across the street. She was standing in her front yard, a toddler tucked under one arm. My father tapped the horn as we passed. The woman waved.

"She was a real firecracker in her day," he said, nodding with sincere appreciation.

"So the appraisal's here in Port?" I said.

"Oh, it's . . ." He trailed off, thinking about something else.

"Dad?"

"It's not so far."

"Out of town then?"

"I guess you could say that."

"Dad."

"Let's just take a little ride and see."

The appraisal, it turned out, was in Belgium, an unincorporated town that was little more than a crossroads. The house was a typical "starter home," small and dark, set too close to the road. Half a dozen houses just like it stretched in either direction. Train tracks passed several hundred feet from the front drive. My father fished the tape measure from underneath the seat, and I grabbed the clipboard. We both got out of the car.

"Nice, level lot," he said.

Petunias grew along the sidewalk leading up to the front door. I could already see my mother's ad: *CHARMING 3BR/1BA in quiet, country setting.*

"Twelve hundred square feet," my father said, guessing. We measured the exterior and found it was exactly that. Inside, the house was vacant. The carpet was faded at the center of the living room, darker around the edges, and you could see where each piece of furniture had been: couch, chair, ottoman, TV console. I caught a faint whiff of septic, which my father had taught me to identify. I noted the lack of storm windows, the electric heat. I waited for my father to tell me, as he always did, that I should never buy anything with electric heat. But he was already measuring the rooms. He flushed the toilets, ran the faucets, checked the fuse box in the kitchen. The linoleum was curling up around the refrigerator. As my father emptied the overflowing drip pan, I stood at the kitchen window, staring past the limp curtains into the tiny, green square of lawn. There was a swing set out there, with dusty furrows beneath each seat, and a sandbox covered with sheets of black plastic.

A thought formed itself in my mind: *this could be your house someday.*

And with that, as if he'd been listening to my thoughts, my father said, "How would you like a house like this?"

The question startled me. "Never buy a house with electric heat," I said automatically.

"But if you were just starting out, though," he persisted. "With a family." There was something like pleading in his voice; he was begging me to listen. I tried to imagine raising children here, watching them play outside on the swings. My husband and I would paint the walls bright colors to hide the imperfections. We'd save money for a new refrigerator. We'd talk about replacing the carpeting.

"I'd be miserable," I said. "I want to play the piano."

"I thought you wanted to be a doctor someday."

We both looked out the window at the empty swings.

"You could go to medical school," my father said, "and become a doctor and then, after you've established a practice someplace, you could cut back on your patient load."

"Why would I want to do that?"

"So you could stay home more. With . . . little ones."

He had really thought this through.

"But what if I don't want children?"

My father turned the faucet on, then shut it off.

"What if I don't want to get married?"

"The washer on this faucet is shot," he said. "See how she leaks?"

"I don't think I want to study medicine anymore."

"She's missing the aerator, too," he said. "That's how come the pressure's so strong." Then, abruptly, he sighed. "I just wonder if there isn't somebody closer than Skokie," he said.

I looked at him. So he had been listening after all.

"My teacher recommended *this* teacher," I said.

My father tamped down the curled edge of linoleum

with his foot, but it sprang right back up again. "Let's get a picture," he said.

Outside, the sun was still strong, though the shadows from the windbreak across the road were lengthening. My father took his old Polaroid Instamatic out of the glove compartment. He shot several pictures of the house from different angles, then spread them on the hood of car, waiting for them to develop.

"You can't make a living playing the piano," he said.

"I could play chamber music," I said. "I could work as an accompanist. I could teach at a university, give private lessons on the side."

My father touched each photograph with his fingertip.

"Or I could just marry for money. Some rich older man."

The corners of my father's mouth twitched upward.

"Which of these pictures do you like best?" he said.

I pointed to the one that showed a peek of the backyard.

"Me, too," he said, and he smiled at me, pleased. And though neither of us said anything more about the lessons, I knew that I would be going to Skokie, if that was what I wanted. *Watch out what you want,* I reminded myself—but no. For once, the words had no power.

I wanted this. I wanted this desperately.

Driving home through the splintering twilight, I watched the ghost-shape of the ranch house fade. Fireflies blazed in the ditches. My life was going to change.

Six

Shortly after I turned fifteen, I decided to break up with my boyfriend, to make more time for my music. Bob was two years older than I was, and very earnest and sweet. I always knew when he was about to kiss me because he'd look left, then right, then left again, as if he were about to cross a busy street. Bob didn't understand why I wouldn't let him drive me to my piano lessons in Skokie. What did I mean, I needed to concentrate? And why wouldn't I come to the phone if he called while I was practicing? I was *always* practicing. Why did I have to be so *disciplined* all the time?

"Practice some other time," he'd say. "I miss you."

We had pulled over by the side of the road somewhere, and I had just noticed that the sharp yellow slice of asphalt lit by our headlights seemed to be, well, *moving*. But it didn't seem like the right moment to bring this up. Billy Joel was singing "Honesty" on Bob's eight-track tape player, and Bob, who was crying, was telling me he would always think of me whenever he heard that song. I said, "But I'm *being* honest," and he said, patiently—he was so *very* patient— "I know that. That's why I said I'll think of you."

"Oh," I said. I had not told him I was breaking up with him because I wanted to be a concert pianist. What I'd told him was that I had decided to become a nun. I'd used the nun story before, at parties on the bluff, when I hadn't wanted to drink or do bong hits or make out with some gross senior I'd never seen before. It was the sort of announcement that took people by surprise. Nobody ever doubted it. It was as if you'd announced you had lice. Everybody just stepped way back.

Bob wiped his nose on his sleeve. I watched uneasily as the asphalt rippled outside my window. It looked like water streaming across the road, only thicker. Deeper.

"So how long have you known?" he finally said.

"Not long."

"Then how can you be sure?"

"I just am," I said, even though the only thing I was sure of right then was that I didn't want to see him looking left, then right, then left anymore. The collar of his letterman's jacket lay heavy across the back of my neck. He was already talking about his class ring, how he wanted me to help him pick it out, how good it would look on my finger. I knew that if we dated for another few months, we'd sleep together. If we slept together for the next two years, we'd get engaged. We'd get married the summer after graduation. Until then, every Saturday night, I'd have to whisper what we'd done together into the dark booth where Father Stone sat like a shadow behind the scrim, his pale ear like a bottomless cup.

"I'm sorry," I said stupidly.

"I need some air," Bob said.

He got out and started to walk, and I opened up my door, too, saying, "Wait."

"What the hell's all over the road?" Bob said.

It was frogs. Thousands upon thousands. The sound was overwhelming. We hadn't heard anything in the car, what with the windows rolled up, and Billy Joel singing about everyone being so untrue.

"Don't move," I shouted to Bob.

"Aw, shit!" Bob said, taking a huge step toward the car. He balanced on one foot, still crying. The underside of his white high-top was dark with goo.

"You're killing them!" I said.

"I can't help it!"

He took another step. Now I was crying, too. The frogs kept coming out of the tall swampy grasses along the roadside, wave after wave, like dark water rising, like a plague sent from the wrathful God in whom we both absolutely believed.

On lesson days, I got to leave my last class early. Nothing could have pleased me more. I waited for my mother at the high school flagpole, in the center of the courtyard, in full view of enough classroom windows to discourage anybody from bothering me. *Dear God,* I'd pray, *let her be on time today, let her get here before the bell rings.* My mother came directly from the elementary school, which let out earlier than the high school, but every now and then she'd get held up by some minor emergency. I'd close my eyes, force myself to keep them closed until I'd counted ten. Likely as not, by the time I peeked, her little red Pinto would be slipping and sliding around the icy circular drive. She'd pull up beside me, lean across the passenger's seat to thump the sticking door.

"How was school?" she'd say, but I'd get in without answering, wait for her to fill the silence. It was only gassing up at the key-pump west of town that I finally started to breathe again, to shed the boiled yellow light of the classroom, to dissolve the wrinkled pit of nervousness that never fully left my chest. Early in my sophomore year

I'd had the misfortune to catch the attention of three members of the wrestling team. Now, they knocked their hips against me if they passed me in the stairwell; they reached into their pants and grabbed themselves when they saw me coming down the hall. After school, I walked home in the street as they trailed me on the sidewalks, chucking small stones and apple cores at the backs of my legs. "We're *coming* for you, sweetheart," they'd call, and then they'd make loud, smacking sounds against the palms of their hands. Raised on stories from the *Lives of the Saints,* stories in which girls were canonized for choosing death over rape, I lived in the fear that I, too, might be forced to choose. And if God decided to test me in this way, I knew that I would fail. I didn't want to die. I wanted to finish high school. I wanted to get into a good conservatory. I wanted . . .

. . . but was hard to imagine what I wanted. I knew only what I didn't want: this school, this dry-throated uneasiness, this feeling I had not yet learned to identify as rage. It was 1980, the year of *giving nippers.* One boy, cheered on by a larger group, would grab an unpopular kid's nipple, twist it hard enough to leave a bruise that—according to locker room wisdom—could give you cancer. I'd gotten a nipper back in September, and the pain had brought me to my knees. Now I was watching that breast anxiously. I had memorized the Seven Deadly Warning Signs.

The two-hour trip to Skokie was a break from all that.

After a day spent holding my arms against my sides, it felt glorious to gesture again, to lift the hood of the Pinto and check the oil and wiper fluid, to reach the squeegee across the windshield while my mother topped off the gas. We made another pit stop, this time for doughnuts and coffee. Then we followed the two-lane highway toward the interstate, accelerating through the sprawl of car dealerships and billboards. We passed the dying farmhouses, dark and still as ghosts; the broken-backed barns; the fundamentalist church. We passed the new subdivisions, with their orderly rows of aluminum prefabs, their identical shrubs and listless trees, their snow-covered flowerpots. Homemade signs promised ANTIQUES 4 SALE; FREE UGLY KITTENS; A TAIL TO REMEMBER TAXIDERMY. A chipped plaster Virgin gazed vaguely at the frozen ground. Nearby stood a wooden cutout of a woman jack-knifed at the waist, fat buttocks pointing at the road.

But as soon as we'd merged onto I-43, the landscape opened like the palm of a hand, fields rising and falling in a gentle undulation like the breathing of a sleeping child. Here were the working dairy farms, each with its various outbuildings, its orchards, its windbreak of pines. Many of the houses had been built from quarry stone, with wide porches and steeply pitched roofs, and the same families had lived in them for generations. My mother told me stories she hadn't heard so much as come to know, stories that spread from person to person the way pollen spreads flower to flower. These stories belonged to the houses in the same way that the houses, the farms, belonged to the land. These stories walked the pastures and slept in the beds and followed the children to school. They were larger, more permanent, than the people who had lived them and, like the people who had lived them, they'd been shaped by the space into which they'd been born: narrow staircases and drafty porches, packed-earth basements and cold root cellars, the crops and the harvests and the winter isolations, the whims of the weather and the clean, wide distance of the sky.

We passed a brick house with a new vinyl addition that sat on its head like a terrible wig. My mother described the woman who had lived there, a woman originally from Chicago. She had been the first person in the county to get linoleum, which she'd ordered not only for the kitchen but the living room as well. Everybody had been invited to see it on the day it was installed: she'd served coffee and pop and sweet chunks of Bundt cake, and people all agreed how very nice it looked. But the woman hadn't known how to care for it, and the following day, she ruined it with floor wax. Within an hour, she'd polished away every last bit of that glorious shine.

Several miles to the south stood another, smaller house with a great front porch tacked across the front of it like a grin. The man who lived there had married a beautiful woman, and this woman had given birth to three daughters, all of whom inherited their mother's golden hair. One night, when the girls were teenagers, the man had come home drunk, raging. He'd had enough of their vanities, he said. He was going to cut their hair, kick the Devil out of their hearts. While he fetched the pinking shears from the woman's sewing basket, she managed to hurry the girls from their bedroom and hide them under the porch. There, shivering in their bathrobes, they listened to their mother's pleadings, the long silence that followed, and when she finally came to get them, she wore a kerchief over her head. The man sobered up and apologized, but the woman's hair never grew back the way it had been. He brought home expensive conditioners, treatments, but the woman passed them along to her daughters instead. He'd been right, she told company as her husband stared into his hands. She *had* been vain. She *was* too old to worry over something as foolish as her hair. It wasn't as if they were youngsters anymore—oh, no, they were finished with all that, you'd better believe it. She was done with all the nonsense that had gone with a pretty head of hair.

This was the landscape my mother painted for me, spreading memory after memory over everything I saw like watercolors over a photograph. Before I knew it, we'd be passing through the suburban sprawl north of Milwaukee, riding the twisting overpasses through the downtown. My mother talked on. Here and there, she'd tighten her grip on the wheel, stopping midsentence if she needed to change lanes, but her voice, when she continued, always was steady, and she'd pick up exactly where she'd left off. I pressed my forehead against the cool window and listened to her voice the way I might have listened to music, following its highs and lows, anticipating its pauses, the inevitable shifts in tone, for my mother spoke to me on these drives the way, some day, she would often speak on our long trips to the Mayo clinic: as if she hadn't spoken to anyone in years. As if she believed she had only the length of this drive, this single journey, to tell me everything she'd learned over the course of a lifetime.

I listened, daydreamed, listened some more. The city streets below the interstate seemed to move like my mother's sentences: long and straight, running parallel to each other without ever actually connecting, punctuated by parking lots and schools, the exclamation points of church steeples straining for the sky. The lake in the distance was pale and empty, a place where anything might be written, unlike the city with its high-rises and clamor, its layerings, its competing obligations. Old cathedrals lifted their chins beside new gas stations; strip malls quarreled with aging Victorians. Boxy brown apartment complexes and condos lined up on the horizon like soldiers on the march. This was an unfamiliar landscape, a language my mother didn't speak. What we saw, we saw literally, with the concrete vision of the eye. Here a house was just a house and not the people who lived there. A bridge was only a bridge and not the story of its crossings.

Perhaps this was why, soon after we'd left Milwaukee behind, my mother's gaze shifted inward. Now she talked about her childhood, about growing up the youngest of nine on the farm she still called *home,* about the way she and her sisters sang as they worked in the massive vegetable gardens, in the orchards, in the family's fields, wearing dresses sewn from cotton feed sacks. She sang on Sundays, too, in the choir loft of Saint Nicholas Church, and she sang to herself at the preserving company, standing beside the conveyor belt, sorting clots of dirt and dead mice and twigs from the produce. She'd started working in the cannery fields the summer before her seventh birthday and, during our trips to Skokie, she took me along with her and her sisters. Mornings before dawn, we waited together, shivering in the early morning chill, for the truck that would shuttle us to the day's work site. She showed me how to fight my way to the outside of the truckbed, where we could hang on to the wooden slats, bracing ourselves for balance. She taught me how to breathe through my mouth to avoid the sick-sweet smell of exhaust. How to duck the streams of tobacco juice that the driver spat from his open window.

"Well, no," my mother said, surprised by my question, "nobody ever fell off the truck because, if they had, they would have been killed." She mused, drifting briefly toward the guard rail, then jerked us back into our lane. "And sometimes we carried knives. We'd have landed on those knives, even if the fall itself hadn't killed us."

And what were the knives for?

"Spinach." My mother bit deep into the word. "When it was in season. But mostly, we picked beans. Penny and a half a pound."

How did the cannery know how much to pay each picker?

"Well, we each had a bucket and our own burlap bag," my mother said. "You picked into your bucket, then emptied the bucket into your bag, and when it was full, you signaled the bean boss to come over with the scale. He'd tie the bag with twine and weigh it right there in front of you. Then he'd punch the weight on your card. You turned in that punch card to get your pay."

Did my mother like the work?

"It didn't matter if you liked it or not because everybody worked all the time. It's just what people did. You didn't even think about it. But I always preferred working outdoors to in, so I didn't mind being a picker. And singing passed the time. We were always singing."

What did they sing?

"Oh, whatever was popular then. The migrants sang too, but they had their own songs, you know, in Spanish."

What were those songs about?

My mother didn't know.

"I should have asked your Uncle Joey," she said one day, a new variation on a story that, by now, I'd heard many times. "He probably could have told me."

Oh?

That particular day it was snowing hard, and the windshield wipers kept freezing to the windshield. Every twenty minutes or so, I'd hold the wheel steady so my mother could roll down the window, lean out, and whack at them with the scraper.

Uncle Joey speaks *Spanish?*

"Well, I assume he does. His people come from Cuba. I guess I never asked."

I thought about Uncle Joey, the first of my uncles I'd been able to tell apart from the others—not because he appeared any different, but because of his laugh. I'd always assumed he was a Luxemburger, like the rest of my uncles, like almost everyone we knew. Had he been a migrant worker?

"Oh, no, he's from Chicago somewhere."

Chicago?! Then how had he met my aunt?

"I honestly don't remember," my mother said. "I was just a little girl. The older ones remember these things, but they don't talk around me."

Why?

"I think it's because of Daddy."

She always drove more slowly when she spoke about serious things, speeding up again as she approached the good parts: punch lines, moments of revenge or revelation.

"It's like we grew up in different families," my mother said. "The older ones had a father; we younger ones never did. I'm the only one who can't remember him at all."

Cars swerved around us, blowing their horns. So many of my mother's memories ended here, with her father's absence, a space I imagined to be smooth and white, like Lake Michigan when it froze over in winter. At the center of all that whiteness was the day of my grandfather's death. He'd been up on a wagon and had lost his balance. He'd fallen and landed on a pitchfork. Where on the farm had this happened? Who had been with him? Where, exactly, was he wounded? Did he die at home or at a hospital? Was he clearheaded? Was he able to tell his family good-bye?

My mother wasn't sure. All she knew was that it had been an accident, nobody's fault.

"But the insurance people ruled it *self-inflicted,*" she said, "because Grandma told them he'd *jumped* off the wagon. If she'd said *fallen,* the insurance would have paid, but English still wasn't spoken much at home, and she didn't know how to explain. Luxemburg was what they all spoke. They say I spoke it, too, when I was very young, before the second world war. Of course, after that, we only spoke English. You didn't want people saying you weren't American."

Jumped instead of *fallen.* I was fascinated by the thought that so much could hinge on the difference of a single word.

"There's one story I've heard about Daddy and me," my mother said, "but I don't know—maybe I made it up. He was lying on the bed, and everybody knew he was dying except me. I crawled up beside him and began to play with my doll. One of my sisters tried to pull me down, but he said, No, let her stay."

Another swerve, another correction. The hum of the tires on the road.

"But that doesn't make sense because later, after I was married, I heard somebody say he died at the hospital. I'd always thought he had died at home. I think I heard that he'd walked into the house after the accident, that it hadn't seemed so bad at first, but I suppose—well, a pitchfork is filthy. They didn't have antibiotics back then. I put a pitchfork through the top of my foot once, right through my boot, when I was eight. I was stacking hay. My foot swelled up like you wouldn't believe."

But I did believe. I could see the foot, pink as quartz, and how my grandmother had to force it down into the steaming pan of Epsom salts. I could see the feed sack dress my mother wore, printed with tiny, yellow flowers. I had watched as she'd chosen this pattern from the pile of sacks at the mill, wondering if her father would have liked it. Wondering what had been his favorite color.

Wondering about the sound of his voice, the sound of his laugh, the way he'd spoken her mother's name.

I could see the room where my grandfather lay dying, forty-two years old with a house full of children, the older ones praying the rosary, the younger ones wide-eyed, confused. I could see the baby on the bed, playing with her doll. I could hear my grandfather's voice: *let her stay.* I felt the emptiness of that bed, where my mother would sleep beside my grandmother until she turned thirteen. The bed where I, too, would sleep as a girl whenever I spent the night. The floury smell of my grandmother's skin. The way she dressed behind the door, facing the wall, as she'd done all those years she'd shared the room with my mother—something I knew long before my mother told me.

Modesty: the first time I saw that word, it claimed the shape of my grandmother's back, the worn gray sheen of her corset. *Chastity:* the nights I lay beside her listening to the chime of the clock, the creak of the walls. *Sorrow:* my body filling the long thin furrow my mother's had made. My grandfather's impression eroded now, lost, nowhere to be found in that bed.

My grandmother's voice in the darkness, soft: Are you awake?

Yes, Grandma, I am.

She presses the warm beads of her rosary into my hand. Whenever I cannot sleep, she says, I pray.

My new teacher, Miss Williams, was in her late twenties. In addition to managing a thriving studio, she was well known as an accompanist. Periodically, she'd cancel several weeks of lessons to go on tour with a singer or violinist, returning with grand stories of the road: lost instruments, horrible pianos, bizarre gifts sent backstage. In her absence I practiced independently, listened to the records she loaned me, and read the biographies of composers and virtuosi she recommended. In particular, I idolized Clara Weick Schumann. Despite undiagnosed pains in her arms, complications from numerous pregnancies, and a husband deteriorating in an asylum, she'd continued to compose and perform. I was fascinated by speculations that she might, after Robert Schumann's death, have married Johannes Brahms. Instead, she'd chosen to devote the rest of her life to music alone.

Did I have such courage? Would I ever dare to sacrifice love for art? Nights, after I'd practiced particularly hard, my arms sometimes woke me with their dull ache. I'd move them around, seeking fresh, cool patches of sheet, and wonder if Clara had done the same thing, listening to the sound of carriages passing over the cobblestones of the Aldstadt. The truth was that I took pride in my painful arms. They were a badge of courage, evidence of my seriousness. Like Clara, I could rise above a trifling thing like pain, and this made me impatient whenever Miss Williams stopped my lessons—at least three times over the course of the two hours we'd spend together—to have me stand, raise my arms over my head, and stretch my neck from side to side. "Every half an hour," she said. "It's important to get in the habit of taking breaks. Set a timer so you don't forget."

Miss Williams had a number of tricks like these. She herself had bursitis in her shoulder, chronic tendinitis in her right pinky finger. After lessons, she'd leave the studio with my mother and me and walk us down the hall to the entryway, where there was a soft-drink machine. My mother would buy two ice-cold cans of Jolly Good Creme Soda, which I'd stuff down the sleeves of my coat, adjusting them until they pressed on the tenderest points of my forearms. Miss Williams, in the meantime, bought her own can, which she held against her neck as we said our goodbyes.

"Hazards of the trade," she said. "You learn to live with such things."

I'd been studying with Miss Williams for nearly two years when she decided to tour full time. Regretfully, she'd no longer be able to teach private students. Tears came into my eyes when she told us this.

"Can you recommend somebody else?" my mother said quickly.

"Yes and no," Miss Williams said.

The woman she had in mind, Evelyn Austin Gall, taught in a nearby suburb. Mrs. Gall, Miss Williams warned, though an excellent teacher, was not the warm and fuzzy type. Now in her fifties, educated in Europe as a child prodigy, she'd had a respectable concert career before marrying late in life and settling down in the United States. We set up an audition in the fall of my junior year.

Mrs. Gall taught out of her palatial home in Highland Park, Illinois. The living room held two grand pianos, a marble fireplace, built-in bookshelves filled with *hardback* books. Ancestral portraits lined the walls. My mother and I had never seen anything like it. Mrs. Gall, it was clear, had never seen anything like either of us: she looked us up and down, taking in our frizzy perms, our unevenly worn shoes and puffy winter coats, our bitten fingernails. Still, she agreed to teach me for a six-month trial period. She suggested that, during that time, my mother park the Pinto in the service driveway. She also hinted that it might be better if we left our shoes at the door. My mother, I noticed, was staring at the bookshelves; I followed the direction of her gaze. There, in plain view, where anybody might see it, was a copy of *The Joy of Sex*.

My mother and I blushed identical shades of pink.

Lessons with Mrs. Gall did not include theory and counterpoint, as they had with Miss Williams. They did include the metronome. Mrs. Gall would set it at one speed, then demand I play at another. If I slowed down or speeded up, Mrs. Gall helped me out by beating the proper time on my shoulder with a flyswatter. She loved to talk about the concerts she'd given at my age, dropping names my mother and I did not know, referring to places we'd clearly never been, praising international restaurants, museums, and galleries we'd obviously never heard of. I left my lessons humiliated, frustrated, embarrassed for both my mother and me, and I retained very little of the excellent critiques she gave, though in college, I'd review the comments she'd written on my music, marveling at her insights, her ingenious fingerings. Several fingering sequences she'd credited to Beethoven himself. When I'd looked skeptical, she'd written out her pedagogical lineage, showing how it had come to her, and from whom. I did not question anything she said to me after that.

But I did not like her any better, did not feel comfortable in her presence. Keeping one eye on that flyswatter, I fumbled and stumbled through pieces that, at home, I could play easily. A few months later, I choked at the regional competition in which Mrs. Gall had entered me, using her highly visible and prestigious name. The harder I tried, the worse everything got. Mrs. Gall, observing the slippery slope of my emotional state, assigned less challenging pieces, but it was no use. I couldn't play for her. I was afraid of her. I couldn't absorb a single thing she said, and it was decided, by mutual consent, that Mrs. Gall and I would part ways.

At my last lesson, she was strangely kind. "Your talent is genuine. If you'd come to me five years sooner . . ." She sighed, then turned to my mother. "When the time comes for college applications, please know I'd be happy to write letters on her behalf."

My mother smiled in the way that meant she was furious.

At the door, Mrs. Gall abruptly kissed me: another surprise. "You just haven't had the opportunities," she said. "But you'll be very successful someday at whatever you do. I am certain of it."

There was genuine goodwill in her eyes, but my mother was not at an angle to see it. Before we reached the car, she stopped me, pulled off her fuzzy mitten, and firmly rubbed the print of Mrs. Gall's lipstick from my cheek.

Knowing what I now know, I see we had many options. There were excellent summer workshops at places like Oberlin and Bloomington; there were boarding schools, such as Interlochen. It is very possible that Mrs. Gall tried to tell us about such things, but the information would have been lost in the general cultural avalanche she released on us each week. And even if I had applied to Interlochen, or a summer workshop, I doubt my parents would have let me go. I was the sort of sixteen-year-old girl who looked like she was twelve, who spent weekends on her grandmother's farm playing Scrabble and working in the garden. I served at church suppers. I dotted my i's with little hearts. Drugs frightened me—I refused a Tic-Tac once at a party, afraid it might be something illegal. Occasionally, one of my friends got hold of a bottle of Tickle Pink, but I wouldn't even take a sip after I'd read that each swallow of alcohol killed millions of brain cells. If I was going to be a concert pianist, I'd need every one.

Mrs. Gall had given us the name of someone at the University of Wisconsin–Milwaukee, a man who no longer performed very much because of crippling arthritis in his fingers. However, neither my mother nor I was eager to take Mrs. Gall's recommendation, and we decided, without ever discussing it, that we'd find another teacher on our own. My mother called every public school music teacher she knew, music directors at Catholic churches, youth orchestras around the Midwest. The name of one teacher kept coming up, a woman at a music conservatory conveniently located in Milwaukee. My first teacher had warned me away from the place, saying it was too large, too commercially oriented. But Miss Williams, who we'd contacted as well, had heard good things about Miss Martinique—though she was surprised to hear Miss Martinique was still teaching.

"She had a number of successful students in the past," Miss Williams said. "But by now she must be in her eighties, at least. I didn't think she was still teaching."

This comforted me. I imagined somebody like Grandma Krier, somebody completely unlike Mrs. Gall. And I liked the idea of Milwaukee. With my new driver's license, I could get there by myself, without inconveniencing my mother. To our surprise, Miss Martinique had openings in her studio schedule. I auditioned and was accepted.

At a glance, Miss Martinique looked about seventy, but when she sat down beside you at the piano, you saw she could easily be a thousand years old. Her skin was the color of a jack-o'-lantern, waxy-looking beneath a truly remarkable layer of base makeup and powder. Whenever she nodded, or gestured with a small, gnarled hand, a powdery aura shimmered all around her. Her auburn-colored wig had tendency to slip, covering one ear. Every now and then she'd poke a long-nailed finger underneath it—*sckritch, sckritch*—and it seemed as if the sound itself, rather than the delicate movement, was what released yet another marvelous cloud of dust. I have no doubt that, in her time, Miss Martinique had been a wonderful piano teacher, but at this point in her life she had forgotten nearly everything she'd ever known about the instrument. Her fingers could no longer function on the keys. She couldn't see well enough to read music. Her vague comments on my scores frequently wandered off the page altogether.

"Lovely, that's quite lovely," was her only comment when, at our first lesson, I sat down and ravaged the first two movements of the Waldstein Sonata. I'd learned them on my own, since leaving Mrs. Gall. Though I'd longed to be told that I played it wonderfully, I knew in my bones that this wasn't so. The piece was too difficult for me. I'd learned it just to be rebellious. I had fully expected to get knocked back down to size.

As I was driving home, two syllables rose into my throat: *uh-oh.*

Each week, Miss Martinique tried to pass our sixty-minute lesson in conversation. How was my trip into Milwaukee? Were the roads all right? And where was it I came from again? And did I have brothers and sisters? Her studio was filled with black-and-white photographs of former students, and soon I knew each of their stories by heart: how long they'd studied with Miss Martinique, what contests they'd gone on to win, which orchestras they'd eventually performed with. I might have half an hour left by the time we got down to the Waldstein. Miss Martinique had seen nothing wrong with assigning the third and fourth movements. She offered no guidance when it came to technique, interpretation, fingerings. "Lovely, that's really quite lovely," she'd said. At the end of each lesson, she'd tell me to "concentrate on your articulation." And that was that.

I knew I was in trouble, but I couldn't bear to admit to my parents how terrible Miss Martinique was, especially after my mother had spent so much time trying to find her. And the drive to Milwaukee was so much easier than going all the way to Chicago. And, frankly, saying I took lessons at a *conservatory* sounded so much more impressive than saying I took lessons in somebody's house or rented studio. The conservatory sponsored frequent recitals, with printed programs to be circulated among relatives and friends, press releases to be sent to the local paper. My parents were pleased with the attention I was getting, proud of the compliments they received on my behalf.

And, last but not least, there was the matter of the grand piano, which my parents had bought for me when I was still studying with Mrs. Gall. The moment she'd heard I was playing on an unreliable upright, not even a reputable Yamaha but some brand she'd never heard of, she nearly melted my poor mother with one of her withering looks.

"No wonder the child is always in pain," she said. "Ruining her fingers on a stiff, uneven keyboard! She must have a decent instrument, something with a lighter action, a consistent touch."

My mother dared to wonder how much a "decent instrument" would cost.

"My dear," Mrs. Gall said to her. "A good piano is not an *expense.* It is an *investment.*"

She called several dealers who, in turn, made several calls, who in turn set us up to see several used pianos. Only a Steinway grand would do, and it had to be built before the Depression, when the construction materials had been first rate. The most appropriate specimens seemed to be stored in Chicago warehouses, and these warehouses were located down in the Loop, where the buildings had boarded-up windows and the streets were strewn with trash. The piano dealers guided my mother and me into huge, creaking service elevators, led us though mazes of stacked furniture, unveiled pianos so massive I wondered how on earth they would fit in our living room. I'd had a shining black instrument in mind, but the one that felt and sounded best was a 1927 Steinway L, with a mahogany body and slightly yellowed, ivory keys. It had been fitted with a device that had turned it into a player piano; you fed what looked like Braille scrolls into a box underneath the keyboard, and the piano, as if by magic, played. Fortunately, this device, coupled with some other cosmetic damage, had made the piano less expensive than others we had seen.

"Excellent," Mrs. Gall said.

By then, my father's real estate company was established, and he'd built several apartment complexes that he managed himself, collecting his own rents, doing most of his own repairs. In the morning, I might see him in suit and tie, heading out for a meeting with the city planner; I might see him in a sports coat, about to take clients to a showing; I might see him in work pants and an old flannel shirt, setting out for a day of roofing, or digging a new sewer line. There was no job he wouldn't do himself if he had the skills to do it, and there were few skills that his years on the farm had not taught him. He worked seven days a week, often twelve hours a day—except on winter afternoons when the Green Bay Packers played.

There was nothing in the hours either he or my mother kept to indicate they'd become financially secure. The son and daughter of farmers, the children of the Depression, they had kept all the habits of people who still hear the wolf outside the door. My mother saved all the slivers of soap and squished them into a lumpy, new bar. My father watered the ketchup until it was pink, the orange juice until it turned pale. The cords of our lamps and appliances looked like snakes after a meal, swollen fat with duct tape. Kids at school made fun of me for wearing the same clothes over and over again. As a child, my mother had only owned one dress, and it had been made from a cotton feed sack—to her, my three sweaters, three shirts, and two pairs of pants (plus my "nice dress" for Sundays and recitals) bordered on what she called "excess." I owned one pair of shoes, plus a pair of gym sneakers. I owned one winter coat, and a light jacket for spring. My brother, being a boy, made do with even less. People, after all, were starving in the world; it was sinful to have too much. My father's car, though well maintained, was still the same old Chevy. My mother's Pinto had no heat and a broken radio.

But when my mother understood that I needed a better piano, she discussed it with my father, who considered it in his abstract way. One day, without warning, he wrote out the check and placed it in my hand.

"The key to doing good work is having the right tools for the job," he said.

The piano took up three quarters of the living room, sprawling there like a Bengal tiger beneath the rummage sale prints, the silvery floral couch inherited from one of my father's tenants. Whenever I thought about what it had cost, I vowed that I would never, in my entire life, ask for anything else again. So what if Miss Martinique was no rocket scientist. At least she didn't hit me with a flyswatter, or rant and rave because I knew nothing about Impressionist painters. Besides, if I abandoned yet another instructor, perhaps my father would think I'd changed my mind, that I wasn't really serious about music, that he and my mother had spent all that money on the grand piano for nothing.

It was a gray afternoon in May, three months since my last lesson with Mrs. Gall. I was butchering a Rachmaninoff étude when the telephone rang. Once, I wouldn't have heard it; now, I leapt up to answer it, eager for the distraction.

"Hello?" I said, crimping the phone between my shoulder and neck so I could rest my arms.

It was Mrs. Gall. She did not bother with preliminaries. She'd happened to run into the teacher she'd recommended for me, the one at the University of Wisconsin–Milwaukee. She was calling to find out why I'd never contacted him. Did I have another teacher?

I did.

Was I happy with this teacher?

I was silent for a moment. Then it all poured out. Mrs. Gall listened, then let me know, in no uncertain terms, how disappointed she was in me. Of course, I must immediately tell my mother about Miss Martinique. Why on earth would I think my mother—or my father, for that matter—wouldn't want to know that something was the matter? Hadn't my poor mother driven me hundreds of miles every week? Hadn't my parents bought me a gorgeous piano? And here I was, wasting my time and their money. I was a junior in high school. Didn't I realize my college auditions were only one year away?

"I'm going to make a few phone calls," Mrs. Gall said, and hung up.

"Who was that?" my mother said, coming into the

kitchen. Then she saw my face. "My goodness! What happened?"

I told her everything.

That night after supper, the phone rang again. I picked it up, cringing, expecting Mrs. Gall. Instead it was a soft-spoken man who greeted me by name, then asked to speak with my mother. His name was Mr. Celeste, and he taught piano at the University of Wisconsin–Milwaukee. He also taught private lessons out of his home, in a suburb only thirty minutes south of Port Washington. He understood from Mrs. Gall that I was looking for a teacher who could help me prepare for college auditions, and he had an opening in his studio.

Would Ann be interested?

I was back on track.

Seven

How *do you discipline yourself?* people asked, but discipline had nothing to do with it. The music I played was like an itch in my throat, a question to be answered, a story to be told. *Discipline:* a word that never entered my thoughts until somebody tossed it into my lap, set me up to walk beneath it as if it were a bucket of cold water. Though sometimes I could hear the word foreshadowed in the tone: *My goodness, Ann, why you are so disciplined? Why do you work so hard?* I'd stare straight ahead, embarrassed, in the same way my friend Dee was embarrassed by her boyfriend, a sweet, strange boy who didn't comb his hair and spoke in a language he'd invented himself.

Even now, it's hard to explain what drew me to the piano with such single-mindedness.

Let's say it is late on a Thursday night, in the fall of my senior year. Let's say I've just finished practicing for the day, so I turn on NPR. Perhaps, tonight, there's a Brahms intermezzo I've never heard before, shimmering in the air like an ornament, an apple, something that was placed there just for me. I've already wiped down the keys and closed the piano lid. I've filled the kitchen sink with cold water, dumped in a tray of ice, and lowered my arms into the soothing chill. Now my arms lay across my lap: humming, satisfied. And yet, I cannot help myself. I move to the piano, finger the keys. Soon, I've managed to rekindle a good portion of the A melody, but the next thing I know, there's my dad in his droopy underwear, blinking at the light, reminding me that there are other people in this house, people who need to get some sleep.

During the night, the scattering of notes I've skimmed arrange themselves into a single idea, a line I can hold in my head like a prayer. In the morning, I comb through this line as I lie in bed, listening to the familiar waking sounds of the house: the thud of the bass from my brother's bedroom, the morning show laughter from the living room, the scrape of a plow going past on the street. The line—I understand this now—is not complex. There's another just beneath it, lumbering and full, bumping up against the surface like a turtle trapped under ice. I am certain I can free it. I only need a few minutes, half an hour, maybe an hour at the most, but school starts at 7:10, early enough so the older kids can work the three to eleven shift, and my father has put his foot down—no piano before seven in the morning or after nine-thirty at night. A rule I understand, even though I resent it. A rule I agreed to a few days after the new piano was delivered.

How people shake their heads at that piano, which cost as much as a good used car. They say that my parents have spoiled me. They say it is no wonder if *that Ann* is too big for her britches, no wonder if *that Ann* always has her nose held up in the air.

That Ann, That Ann, like a first and last name.

I rise, shivering in the icy room, and kneel on the carpet to say my morning prayers. I am seventeen, and so I do crazy things like sleep with my window open. I deny myself: the best seat, the first choice, the biggest piece. I turn the other cheek. At school, it's a sport to tease me, trip me, knock my books out of my hands, because everybody knows I won't tell, and I don't have a boyfriend to protect me. Am I too big for my britches? Do I have my nose in the air? These are the complaints my teachers have made: to me, to my parents, to the other kids who agree. It's a terrible thing, to believe you're good at something. To believe that you could be, for heaven's sake, a *concert pianist.* Who ever *heard* of such a thing? Where does *that Ann* get these fine ideas?

Here comes the queen, one of my teachers likes to say. *Make way for the queen.*

I take my seat, arrange my books, pretend I do not hear.

My piano teacher, Mr. Celeste, has told me all about the Greeks, how they believed that music had the power to transform the human soul. I desperately hope this is true. I probably *am* too big for my britches. I probably *am* arrogant, vain. And then there is my mind, which is often unruly. Thoughts fly into my head that are so frightening it is easier to pretend they are not mine. One day, I passed the antique crucifix in the hall between my bedroom and my parents'—the one my mother took down to show me when I was very young, explaining how to unlatch the back, take out the blessed candles, the scroll with instructions for Last Rites—and, for some reason, it caught my eye as if I'd never seen it before. As I studied the agonized line of Christ's mouth, it occurred to me that I was looking at, well, a dead guy, and that he was hanging in the middle of my house, and that this was as weird as the weirdest thing I'd ever read about in *National Geographic*. In fact, we had the most remote populations beaten, hands down. I saw that everything was simply a matter of perspective, meaningful or meaningless according to custom alone. I took the crucifix off the wall and buried it under the towels in the linen closet. The next day, it was back on the wall.

My mother looked at me funny for days.

Without music, without the line that now plays in my head, I am certain such thoughts would overwhelm me. The tidy truths that have formed my life, like the neatly shaped hedges around my house, would be mowed down, torn away. And then there would be no point to anything—would there? There would be no reason to pray, to get out of bed, to move through the day. There would be only the chlorine smell of the shower, the yellow quiver of eggs on my plate, the chill puddle of dread in my stomach at the thought of another school day. The green tile lining the corridors, voices cut by the razor-slash of locker doors, the tin-whistle shriek of the school bell, the crackle of daily announcements read by giggling seniors over the intercom. Even these sounds can be transposed, rearranged into an indifferent song that shields me as I slip out of homeroom to the drinking fountain, which I call a *bubbler,* to linger as long as I can. As I rush down the steps that lead to the locker rooms while the boy who insists even teachers call him Boner steps on my heels, shouting, "Flat tire!" as I enter the sprawl of the cafeteria with its pounding jukebox, its stale odor of American cheese.

Lunch is at 11:10. Too early for anybody to be hungry, but we all shovel it in. I slide my tray in at the edge of the table where my friends sit dipping tater tots into a substance Ronald Reagan has declared a vegetable. These friends are good people: I know this. These friends are much better people than I am. They are firmly grounded in the world. The girls talk about their diets; the boys tease the girls, speak in shrill, falsetto voices. The popular kids call them "art-fags." I am an art-fag, too. It is a relief to be something, even an art-fag. It's a relief to rest at the edge of this group of friends who sign their notes "love always" and who, for the most part, after graduation, I'll never see again.

I try to pay attention, try to laugh when a boy throws a perfectly aimed tater tot down the front of a girl's shirt. It *is* funny. It is also not there. I am not there, distracted as I am, working the line like a needlepoint, in and out, up and down, revealing it piece by piece. My first teacher taught me to play music by ear. My next teacher, Miss Williams, taught me to memorize music by reading it and hearing it in my head. My new teacher, Mr. Celeste, gives me articles by sports psychologists showing that athletes who think through their actions—not as observers, watching themselves, but as if they are actually experiencing their movements—excel over those who do not. I am teaching myself to practice this way. I re-create the sounds I have heard, transcribe them onto the page. I see the notes before my eyes, feel the keyboard under my hand.

Lunch is over by 11:35, and as I separate my paper products, my silverware, I realize that I can't bear to face the afternoon. I tell a friend that I feel sick, that I'm going to head home—would he tell my biology teacher? My friend rolls his eyes.

"What should I tell him this time?" he says. "The intentional flu?"

"Rabies," I say, and I bite him on the neck.

"Bitch," he tells me pleasantly. The other kids think we are sleeping together, a deception that benefits us both. He is a homosexual. (We pronounce the word seriously, diligently, emphasizing all the syllables.) And I—well, I'm not sure what I am. Maybe some kind of eunuch. After all, I could have dates, but I turn them down. Turn up my nose, the other kids say. It will serve me right if I never get married. It will serve me right if I spend the rest of my life alone. Only music can save me. Only music has the power to transform my soul. Dimly, I am aware that it is prayer—devotion to Christ—that I should be endowing with these magical properties. But prayer leaves me feeling anxious, leaves me feeling that no matter how hard I try, God will find me wanting. I am neither bad nor good but something in between. I am what the Bible calls *lukewarm.* I am what God will spit from His mouth.

I collect my coat from my locker, where somebody has scrawled WET DREAM in thick black permanent marker. Perhaps it is the same person who has been shoving notes through the vents, saying that he is going to give me the bloody fuck I need, stuck up cow, you better watch your step. In the pocket of my coat, I've tucked a paring knife I have pilfered from the kitchen; in my purse, I keep a slender bottle of pepper spray I ordered in secret from a catalogue. Who is writing these notes? It could be anybody. The wrestlers who made my sophomore year hell have all graduated, gone off to who knows where. Perhaps it's the boy who sits behind me in art class, bragging about how he and some friends broke into an elderly woman's apartment one night. "I don't know why she was crying," he says, laughing. "All we wanted was for her to cook us some eggs. But she was fuckin' crying so hard she kept dropping them on the floor." It could be the boy who, at a bluff party in September, teased and twisted and dragged a girl who liked him into the bushes, forced his way into her one hundred feet from the open trunk of the car where the rest of us had gathered to drink beer. Later, I found her sitting in my mother's car. Please, she begged, don't say anything. Please just take me home. It could be a member of the basketball team, which has pledged to beat up the school's single black male student—a transfer who has just started school that fall—if he thinks about looking at a white girl. It could be the anonymous figure who jumped my friend Dee's boyfriend in the park one night, calling him queer, leaving him with cracked ribs and a broken jaw.

Weekends I work at my parents' real estate office, where potential buyers from Milwaukee talk about how they want to move to a small town for their kids, for the safety, for the good schools, and I wonder what on earth they are talking about. But then, I often feel this way. There is the surface of things—the shining lake, the church on the hill, the sweet-faced women in the downtown shops—and then there is the way things are. There is the little town with its clean, well-lit streets—and then there is the knife in my pocket. The God who is Love—and the God who condemns homosexuals, people of other faiths, people who have abortions or use birth control, people who have sex outside of marriage, people who get divorced and remarry. The single, sanguine story everybody agrees to tell—and the stories like my own, trapped beneath that stifling weight.

Who frightens me more—the boy who writes me these terrible notes, bearing down so angrily that I can trace the impression of his letters, understand their meaning, with my fingers? Or the God who, like the boy, is bent on controlling me, keeping me in my place, keeping my mind on Him? *Better watch your step.* If only I can make it until Christmas break. If only I can make it through the six weeks after that, when my first round of college auditions begins. If only I can do well enough to get into a good conservatory. If only I can survive until August, without something terrible happening.

If only. *Da-DEE-dum.*

That Ann. DA-DA.

It is familiar, it is Brahms. The line is back in my head.

I slip out of the school by a side door, cross the athletic

field. The chill licks away the fog of the classrooms, the overheated hallways and dull, fluorescent lights. Heading north on Holden Street, I pass the neatly kept houses, the snow-covered, geometric lawns. Christmas trees twinkle in every front window; lights hang in crisp, bright strings from the porches and mailboxes. A plastic Santa glows on a rooftop, holding up an arrow that points to the chimney. I am starting to feel better. I will make hot chocolate and work on the intermezzo, sounding it out until three o'clock, the hour I usually start to practice. Then I will switch over to what I should be working on, my audition pieces: the Bach suites, the Chopin ballade, the Beethoven sonata, the Bartók variations. At my lesson tomorrow, I'll tell Mr. Celeste about the intermezzo, play what I've been able to come up with. He will grumble a bit before rising, combing his bookshelves for the music. *This is dessert,* he will say, tucking it into my satchel. *After the Beethoven. After the broccoli and carrots.*

I will make it till Christmas. I will make it to the end of the school year. Tonight, I will tell my mother, *I took another sanity day,* and she will write my excuse on a piece of the thick, creamy stationery she receives from her own students every year, along with the bottles of perfume, the fruitcakes, the knickknacks, and homemade ashtrays.

Of course, there is another side to all this. There is the part of my life that is neither school nor church, the part that I love, the part that I sense I will lose for good if I ever step out of its rhythms. There is my maternal grandmother's kitchen, and her hundred-acre farm, and the gentle swell of fields, fringed with woodlands. There is the color of the landscape, the tans and browns and winter-whites, the spectacular greenness of springtime. There is my mother and father. There are my uncles and aunts, cousins and second cousins, the hearty clamor of reunions and holiday suppers, Grace that swells like a symphony: *Bless us O Lord and these Thy Gifts.* There is the shared language of absolute faith, the shared reason of people who have lived out their lives within twenty miles of the place where they were born, the land beneath them like the heart of a single organism, a vast and powerful drum. There is the comfort of such numbers, the ease of being swept along with the tide, of giving yourself over to the seasons of marriage and birth, and birth, and birth, grandchildren and great-grandchildren, land and a house and a garden behind it, a kitchen like my grandmother's, humming like a hive.

Where does the piano fit into all this? The hours I spend practicing, or listening to music, or talking with Mr. Celeste about composition, theory, the Greeks? I imagine Orpheus attempting to transform my grandmother's soul with his lyre. She stares at him hard, neither friendly nor unfriendly. She says, Are you supposed to be a boy or a girl? She says, When you finish up your racket there, run down the road and tell Uncle Joe to bring his gun, there's another opossum trapped in the silo.

Discipline means nothing to my grandmother either. Discipline is simply the way you live your life. You don't sit down until your work is finished, whatever that work might be, and your work will not be finished till God calls you to the grave and, if you're lucky, lets you rest a while before He dreams up something else for you to do. My grandmother isn't sure what to think about my music. She believes it is a gift from God. She also believes that it's something that could lead me away from home and into trouble. I am her godchild, her particular responsibility. I am also the oldest child of her youngest child, her baby's baby. Her love for me is as concentrated, as rough and raw as a cat's tongue. I squirm beneath it, half in pleasure, half in pain.

"Music is the language of angels," she says in the same tone she'd use if she saw me about to squirt lighter fluid directly into the burning barrel. The tone she'd use if something I'd said came close to disrespect of the Church.

It is the day of Christmas Eve. I am sitting at my grandmother's table while she stands frying doughnuts at the stove. As I peel withered apples from the bucket I've hauled up from the root cellar, two little girl cousins sit across from me, licking their fingers. Each time my grandmother lifts another doughnut from the crackling grease, it's their job to fetch it, shake it in a bag of sugar, then arrange it, still warm, on a plate. The air simmers with the burnt, sweet smell of frying dough. More cousins are playing on the floor with a cigar box full of dominoes. They stand them on end, arrange them in precarious lines, argue over who gets to knock the first one down. "Jeez!" they say, and "Youse guys!" and "Cut it out, once!" In the rocking chair, a cousin just two years older than I am is nursing her second child. Her first crawls around on the floor, menacing the dominoes, but the older children push him patiently aside, as if he is a windup toy instead of a beautiful, tow-headed boy. My second cousins all seem to be beautiful tow-headed children. All I would have to do is graduate, and get married, and produce a beautiful tow-headed boy like this one, and it would mean more to my family than any scholarship I might win, any concert career I might achieve, more than any other single thing I might ever do with my life.

There are shouts from the living room, where my uncles and older male cousins are watching sports on TV. The house cat rockets in, wild-eyed; the crawling baby abandons the dominoes and motors after him, chiming, *Kee! Kee!* One of my aunts is making another batch of dough; another aunt washes lunch dishes; another aunt is making a pot of Maxwell House Coffee, vaulting the children, the cat, the dominoes on her way to the sink. My mother has taken the trash outside to the burning barrel. From the window, I can see her at the edge of the bean field, the black plume of smoke rising—so it seems—from the top of her head like a feather. She feeds the fire slowly, adding to it piece by piece. To her right is the outhouse attached to the chicken coop; to her left is the double shed. Beside that stands the old corncrib where my brother and cousins and I played jail. There's the milk house and the barn with its double silos. There's the cow pen, empty now, the barbed-wire fence coming loose, and the steeple of Saint Nicholas Church, poking through the dark line where the fields meet the sky.

My mother and I have been here since early this morning, helping with Christmas preparations. Tomorrow, the house will fill with over a hundred people, families arriving to eat the noon dinner in shifts, others arriving for the evening meal, everyone bringing a dish to pass. In addition to the kitchen table, where twenty-odd people can sit, there will be card tables in the living room for the young people, an oilcloth spread on the kitchen floor for the children, everybody eating on paper plates and drinking from plastic cups. There will be dollar bills for the grandchildren, fifty-cent pieces for the great-grands; there will be Secret Santa exchanges, fruitcakes and pfefferneusse, homemade Christmas tree ornaments, wreaths, candles, pinecones rolled in glitter. There will be a pile of coats on my grandmother's bed that reaches halfway to the ceiling. All day, children will sneak into the bedroom to tunnel into the middle of those coats, just the way I once did. All day, there will be the slamming of doors, the rasp of coats coming off and going on, the crying of babies and the fussing of children, the hearty laughter of the men, the peals of outrage and delight from the women, the clatter of plates, and the sound of the television.

I have finished the bucket of apples, and now I set down the paring knife, rest. Any kitchen task like this—chopping onions, slicing bread, peeling apples—bothers my wrists and arms, but I don't want to say anything. It would look like I'm just being lazy. It would look like I'm trying to get out of work. And isn't it true that even when I hurt, I still manage to play the piano at least three hours a day? The house cat slinks down from the windowsill, wriggles in beside me on the long wooden bench my grandfather made. He rubs his broad flat face against my sleeve as if he is a kitten instead of the big, bad broken-eared tom he is. I scratch his chin. My wrist aches.

"Have the barn cats been fed?" I ask.

My grandmother looks up from the stove, a quick, fond glance I understand. She leaves these little tasks for me—feeding the barn cats, gathering eggs—because she knows how much I enjoy them. Knows that, like my mother, I enjoy working outdoors.

In the refrigerator, there's a Tupperware container full of multicolored scraps: Jell-O, the dried-out heel of a roast, stale potato chips, leftover breakfast cereal, sour milk. I carry it out to the entryway, stepping over my cousins, the dominoes, the baby. In the chilly bathroom by the stairs to the basement, I add a few scoops of cat chow from the fifty-pound bag my grandmother gets at the mill. My coat hangs on a peg by the door; I put it on, step outside into the sudden silence of a vast cathedral. The cold is stunning. Radiant. My eyes smart and tear. Snow has erased the roof of the barn, the shed, the milk house. The winter sky presses down, the color of smoke, and I smell the burning barrel as I follow the partially shoveled path toward the barn, follow the harsh rasp of my sneakers. Somewhere, a crow coughs. A loose shingle flaps. Around me, the fields hold the absolute weight of sleep, fringed by yellow stubble, a few dark clots of earth.

A word shapes itself in my mind: *holy.* It splits the crude shell of the word I've been taught and emerges, shimmering and whole. God is here, in these dormant fields, in the bald-headed woods beyond. God is in the crow's call, and the watery shadows cast by the barn. God is in my restlessness. God is in my love of this place and my fear that I will never find the courage to leave it, that it will smother me gently and sweetly and indifferently, like a sleeping parent rolling over upon a child. God is in the thrum and hush and spin of the world beyond. God is a moment like this one: reverent, transcendent, when the very air seems to shine.

The barn door is frozen shut. I bump it hard with my hip, jump back. Icicles fall from the eaves like diamonds shattering at my feet. Now the heavy door slides just enough for me to slip inside. *"Kitty-kitty-kitt-eee,"* I say, imitating my grandmother's call. The barn is silent, empty except for the pigs grunting softly in the adjoining lean-to, the rattle of mice in the grain bins. I remember how an aunt once led me out to the barn on Christmas Eve, back when I was small enough to need to hold her hand. There were dairy cows then, and their sweet grassy smell; there was a bull with a ring in his nose. My aunt had promised me that at midnight, the animals would speak, and when I said I didn't hear anything, she said, well, it wasn't midnight yet, so they were probably still thinking about all the things they wanted to say.

"Kitty-kitty-kitteee!"

Now I feel them watching from the rafters, from the top of the steps leading to the second floor where the machinery is stored. I dump the Tupperware's contents into an old pie tin, fill the other with snow from the drift beneath the broken windows. The cats appear like ghosts, eyes aglow in the dusky light. They dance forward and back until I step away from the food. Then they surge forward, a dozen or so. I recognize an orange tabby, a dirty white tom with a missing eye. There's a new one with a tail shaped like a crank, broken in at least two places. A tiger-stripe rubs against my legs, but flinches when I stoop to pet her. She darts out of reach, then rolls and rolls in a pile of loose straw.

It's a far cry from a storybook manger with its clean, yellow straw, its fluffy white sheep. Cobwebs hang in dirty clots from the crossbeams. Breadlike clumps of old manure fill the troughs. The barn cats growl and purr, tails lashing; the ceiling groans with every gust of wind. Still, it is Christmas Eve. I am a child again, clinging tight to my aunt's mittened hand. I am waiting for the animals to speak, believing, for this moment, that they can.

We spend Christmas Eve with Grandpa and Grandma Ansay, the way we do every year. My mother invites them over for a six o'clock supper, something simple, for my grandmother doesn't care for rich foods. Afterward, as the broiler pan soaks in the sink and the odor of chicken settles everywhere, we all sit around the Christmas tree and begin, one at a time, to open Christmas presents. It's an awkward time because my father never gives anybody anything—though my mother always hopes it will be otherwise. My grandparents give everybody the same thing: one-hundred-dollar U.S. savings bonds. As my brother and I open my mother's gifts, my grandmother laments the cost, the waste, the excess. "Oh, say!" she says at my new pair of boots. "Too much, too much!" The stroke has robbed her of all but a few phrases. She pokes my grandfather until he opens the single gift my mother has addressed to them both, then peers into the box of chocolates as if it contains tarantulas. "Oh, say!" she says, laughing unhappily. But—as my mother well knows—my grandfather loves chocolate, and he is a man who does not love much. Love has been worked out of him, toiled out of him. Even in retirement, his hands are splayed with monstrous yellow calluses. When he takes the first piece of chocolate, tucks it under his mustache, my grandmother slaps at his hands. He ignores her, takes another. She slaps harder. She hits him as hard as she can, limp-wristed, flailing. He makes a swift, rough gesture and their knuckles click.

"G'wan," he says.

She says something nobody understands, but my grandfather says, "That's enough."

It's time to distribute my presents: an antique teacup for my mother's collection, a sweater for my brother, matching pillow shams I've sewn for my grandparents' beds. Because the pillows shams are homemade, my grandmother lets them pass. My grandfather, bright-eyed with sugar, pats them with a massive hand. I don't give my father a gift because, if I do, he'll simply return it. He does this even if somebody gives him something he really needs, something he'd buy for himself. Or else he'll refuse to open it. He'll joke about it, urge us to open it ourselves, then set it on a shelf to open "later." It will stay there for several days, several weeks. One day, we'll glance at the shelf and discover it is gone.

This year, my brother has gifts for everyone, too, and this is unexpected because lately, like my father, he has shied away from gift-giving, from family events, from emotion. At fifteen, a loose-boned shrug has become his sword; selective deafness his shield. Now, he seems like his younger self again, eager and sweet-natured. For my grandparents, he has made a towel holder in the shape of a frog. My grandmother is delighted with this. For my mother, there's is a floral coffee mug with her name on the side, and a bag of coffee beans to go with it. My mother flushes, proud and pleased. For me, there's an adjustable ring, mounted with a circular frame in which a little round-eyed girl holds a little round-eyed kitten. I love this ring. It is exactly what I'd have chosen for myself. I put it on my finger, squeeze to make it fit. "Thanks," I say—everybody says—impressed, but my brother isn't finished. It seems he has a gift for Dad, who is already laughing, waving it away, asking, "Did you keep the receipt?"

"You have to open it," Mike says. "Once you open it, you can have the receipt."

Mike wears his hair long so that it covers his eyes. He

pushes the gift at our father's chest, then steps away, so that Dad has to grab it to keep it from falling. "If you break it, Dad," Mike warns, "you won't be able to take it back."

The gift makes an oddly musical sound when our father turns it over in his hands. Now everybody is curious. Dad stands up and sits down and stands up again, and then he tells my brother *he* should open it. "*You* open it," my mother tells my father, giving him a no-nonsense look, which inspires my grandmother to cry, "Too much, too much!" which means she is taking my father's side, which means that now my father *has* to open it to save face. He sits. We all watch as he loosens the tape, peels away the wrapping paper carefully, so that it can be reused.

There in a tall, thin glass jar, rolling around in the murky water, are a dozen flesh-colored balls.

Testicles?

For a moment, nobody says anything. Mike waits, his long hair curtaining his eyes.

"What's this?" our father quavers, holding out the jar for my mother to read. "What does this say?"

My mother sounds out the words on the bright orange label: *Gefilte* fish. None of us have ever heard of such a thing. None of us can imagine where he might have gotten it.

"Fish balls," Dad says, too heartily. "Well. How very nice."

My brother says, "Do you want the receipt?"

For a moment, we all imagine Dad carrying the fish balls back into the store where they were purchased. We have seen him return just about everything: half-eaten foods that weren't quite right, umbrellas, towels, clothing, even a two-year-old pair of shoes that had been "guaranteed to last a lifetime." But can he go through with this?

"Uh," he finally says. "No. I think this is something I better keep."

A shadow of a smile plays around the corners of my brother's mouth.

In fact, everybody is smiling now, even Dad, and I finally release my breath, thinking, Well, that wasn't so bad. But thoughts like this only tempt the gods. After the wrapping paper has been folded and saved for next year, my father suggests a little piano music, a recital, how about it, Pumpkin? My grandfather has been dozing in a sweet sugar coma, but now his eyes fly open with alarm. "Play! Play!" chimes my grandmother, knowing how my grandfather will hate it. "I'll be right there," Mom sings from the kitchen, where she's doing something wonderfully aggressive to the broiler pan. Mike is halfway out of the room, but the old man is quicker. "Hold up there, Tiger," Dad says, jiggling the jar of gefilte fish. "Let's listen to the Pumpkin play."

The Pumpkin doesn't want to play any more than the Tiger wants to listen, but I sit down at the piano anyway and begin, cruelly, the first of the Bartók Opus 20 improvisations. It will be another hour before my grandparents finally go home, another three hours before my mother and brother and I will put on our coats and head to Midnight Mass, where we'll take turns nodding off between shrill bursts from the aging choir. Bartók is perfect for a moment like this. It is every word I've been holding back since my grandparents stepped through the door. It's my father's jolly refusals to open his gifts, the mysterious hurt this masks. It's my mother's hand-to-hand combat with the broiler pan. It's my brother's brief sphinx of a smile. It's the round-eyed girl holding the kitten, and the round-eyed girl who wears that image on her finger, trying to live up to all that it suggests even as she knows she cannot. Eight variations. Eight states of mind. I relish the dissonance, the irregular meter; I flatten my fingers to achieve an even brassier, percussive tone. I am into this now, it's no longer a recital, I have disappeared and something wild and wordless is shining in my place like fire. When I finish the final improvisation and rise, lending the weight of my body to the final chord, I can't quite remember how I came to be in this room.

Then I see the faces of my family, the glazed-over eyes, the open mouths. They look like people who have been tied down and beaten. I meant to play only the first few improvisations. Somehow, I have performed them all.

Nobody applauds.

"Maybe," my mother says faintly from the doorway. "A Christmas carol . . . would be nice?"

A Christmas carol. I melt down onto the bench. Humbly, I begin to play "Silent Night" in slow, block chords. I can feel the mood in the room begin to change. My father uncrosses his arms and legs. My mother actually takes a seat. When my grandfather slips the last of the chocolates from the box, I wait—watching from the corner of my eye—for my grandmother to slap him, but she doesn't. She has pulled herself forward on the couch, and when I begin the second stanza, breaking into a few light arpeggios, she astonishes us all by beginning to sing.

Stille nacht, heilige nacht
Alles schläft, einsam wacht

I remember, vaguely, my grandmother's voice before the stroke, before she became the person she is now, locked into the straitjacket of her body, locked into a faith that offers her no comfort, locked into a marriage that should have ended long ago. My grandmother's voice is not beautiful, but it is true, and the words she cannot speak roll like a miracle off her tongue. Now my mother is singing, too, in her thin soprano, and there's my father's wavering baritone.

My brother doesn't sing, but he does shake the hair out of his eyes while my grandfather rolls the last morsel of dissolving sweetness around on his tongue.

I play on and on, verse after verse. I am overwhelmed with love for my life, for everyone in this room. It is exactly as the Greeks foretold. The artificial Christmas tree shines.

Eight

I sat on the examination table, shivering in the white paper gown. I had strep throat again, I knew it, even without the throat culture. One of the things I liked about our family doctor was that he listened when you told him these things. He was tall and stooped and handsome, in a quiet way, and if you weren't feeling well, he looked genuinely sorry to hear it.

There was a knock on the door. "Oh, no," Dr. Melchek said, coming into the room. "Not you again."

"Oh, yes."

I'd had strep throat off and on for over a year. I hadn't really minded it because it meant that I could stay home from school. But this was different. It was August; I'd graduated from high school in June. I'd been accepted at the Peabody Conservatory, and I was supposed to leave for Baltimore in just a few more days.

"How's the piano-playing?" Dr. Melchek said, as he swabbed out my throat.

"Fine," I said, trying not to gag.

My Peabody audition had been a series of firsts: my first time seeing the Atlantic Ocean, my first time in a taxicab, my first time exposed to people my age who were as focused on their music as I was. Students came to Peabody from all over the world, and I listened to the jostle of languages in the corridors—Mandarin Chinese, Polish, Portuguese—the way I might have listened to a twentieth-century composer, alternately wincing and wondering at the unexpected sounds. Even English sounded different here, seasoned with Spanish, Yiddish, Korean. Outside the Conservatory walls, in the streets, I heard native Baltimore voices, liquid sounds and singing tones. I luxuriated in new diphthongs, in fresh highs and lows, marveled at the way people called to each other, multisyllabic names ringing out like bells. I saw yarmulkes and dreadlocks; I saw saris and African robes. I ate grape leaves and gyros, curries and egg rolls, steaming platters of crab legs, bagels encrusted with poppy seeds and salt. Three weeks later, when the acceptance letter came, I'd canceled my remaining auditions and started to pack right then and there. Much to my mother's amusement, I kept the open suitcase at the foot of my bed, and this is what I lived out of—leaving my dresser drawers empty—until it was time to leave for Maryland.

"How are your arms holding up?" Dr. Melchek asked.

I held them out. He pressed his thumbs up and down the length of my forearms.

"Any tenderness?"

I shrugged. "A little."

"Do the ice baths help?"

I nodded. Twice a day, I emptied the ice tray into the kitchen sink, then filled the basin and submerged my arms. After recitals, when no ice was handy, I did my soda pop routine, buying a couple of cold cans and stuffing them down my sleeves. My arms were fine. Or, at least, they weren't any different than they always were. Sometimes they burned. Sometimes they buzzed. Other times they were silent.

"Anything else?" Dr. Melchek said.

I hesitated. My mother had wanted me to mention my legs, but I felt stupid bringing it up. It wasn't something that happened very often. Just once in a while, like after I went jogging two days in a row, or climbed the steep hill that led from the downtown to Saint Mary's Church. A few hours later, my legs would start to burn. Just like my arms, when I practiced too much. It didn't always happen, and it never lasted more than a day or so. It always went away.

Dr. Melchek waited.

"My legs hurt sometimes after I run," I said.

He pressed his thumbs along my shins, the way he'd done with my arms. "Anything?" he asked.

"Nope," I said.

Dr. Melrose raised his eyebrows. "Try more walking and less running," he said.

"OK."

I was eager to get the prescription and go. I didn't want him to think I was one of those people who was always sick, always convinced that something was wrong, someone like Grandma Ansay. Of course, something *was* wrong with my grandmother—she'd never regained full use of her right side after the stroke, and her speech was garbled, exhausting—but everyone seemed to think she might have overcome these things, if she'd done her physical therapy, if she'd tried a little harder. At any rate, she only made things harder on herself, shutting herself away. People felt sorry for her, but they got annoyed with her, too. It wasn't as if she couldn't do *anything*. She could watch television, for Pete's sake. She could read. She could go out onto the patio, take in a little sunshine, instead of sitting indoors all the time.

On my way home from Dr. Melchek's, I stopped in to see her one last time, careful to conceal my prescription deep inside my backpack. No one in my family had ever caught one of my strep infections, but I knew that if my grandmother found out I was sick, she'd develop a sore throat on the spot.

The house was dark, the curtains drawn. I rang the bell, waited, rang the bell again. My grandfather answered the door when he was home, but he spent as much time as he could out of the house, playing cards at the senior citizens' center. Guiltily, I hoped that my grandmother would decide it wasn't worth the bother of getting up, but after several minutes, she appeared at the door.

"Come, come," she said, motioning me to follow her through the foyer into dark, stale air. When I snapped on the lamp beside her parlor chair, I saw that she was crying, had been crying, perhaps, for most of the day. This was not unusual. My grandmother's grief was endless. Now she continued to weep, her rosary pooled in her lap, as I chattered about the courses I expected to take at Peabody, the letter I'd gotten from the girl who would be my roommate, steadfastly ignoring her tears the same way that my grandfather and parents did. If you asked her what was wrong, it only made her cry harder, and what was the point of that? If you asked her where it hurt, she'd say, "Hurt! Hurt!" and wave her good hand up and down the length of her body—an accusation, a strange benediction, I did not want to know which.

The Peabody Conservatory stood directly across from the George Washington Monument in Charles

Square, a once-grand historic neighborhood that had been swallowed up into Baltimore's sprawling red light district. The Conservatory itself was a physical haven—nicknamed, affectionately, *the cloister*—enclosed by gates and a high stone wall surrounding a private courtyard. The entrance was monitored by security guards and video cameras but, from time to time, an intruder still managed to slip through. Whenever this happened, the resident assistant, a dark-eyed flutist nearly as slender as her instrument, ran up and down the halls telling us to stay in our rooms with the doors locked. Outside, drug dealers lounged on the bus stop benches; panhandlers stood on the corners, rattling cups. If they didn't like the looks of you, they'd follow you for blocks, alternately wheedling and cursing.

My first week at the Conservatory, a man offered me money for sex. I'd been returning from the Korean market a block away from campus. It was midmorning; the streets were filled with people. When he said hello, I did what I would have done in Port Washington: I smiled, returned his greeting. The next thing I knew, he was pressing a wad of bills into my palm, trying to steer me toward the open car door where two of his friends sat waiting. His touch wasn't rough, but brotherly, cajoling, as if we were playing a game. "Sir?" I said, not wanting to be rude, worried that I might be overreacting. "Excuse me, sir?"

Then I woke up. I dropped the money and took off running and I didn't stop until I'd dashed through the gates of the Conservatory, where the security guard dozed over his gun, across the main courtyard and through the cafeteria and up the back stairs to the third floor of the women's dorm. There, I burst into my room and gasped, "A man offered me money to get in his car!"

My roommate, Leigh, looked up with interest. "How much?"

"That's not the point," I said.

"Did you keep it?"

"Of course not!"

Leigh sighed dramatically. Her face assumed the expression of a world-weary parent. "You spoke to him, right?" she said.

I could not deny it. "He spoke to me first."

Another sigh. "What did I tell you about making eye contact? Do we have to go over this again?"

Leigh was a soprano. She'd already found a boyfriend, a bass player who liked to walk on the furniture in the dormitory lounge, pretending he was the Pink Panther. They'd met at a party during the first week of classes. "You look like a television," he'd told Leigh, "the way you turn on and off." That was it, they had fallen in love—despite the general disapproval of everyone in the women's dorm. How could Leigh make time for a relationship without cutting into her singing? What would happen down the road, when their careers pulled them different ways? We were all, I think, a little in love with Leigh ourselves. She had long dark hair and button-black eyes, perfect pitch and an impressive Grateful Dead collection. Her hobbies included riding motorcycles and dressing up in period costumes to attend Revolutionary War reenactments. And me? I had no hobbies. Sunday mornings, I went to Mass at Saint Ignatius, the little church around the corner and, during the week, I lit candles at the grand Basilica across from the city library. Every morning, I rolled out of bed and onto my knees, where I made the sign of the cross and said an Our Father and a Hail Mary. I did these things automatically, unselfconsciously, the way I brushed my teeth and combed my short, overpermed hair. Why they'd paired the two of us as roommates was beyond me, but I was endlessly grateful. Leigh looked out for me, and I clung to her as if she were a Sherpa guide.

Now she put up one graceful finger, warning me to wait, and left the room. Within a minute, she was back with Susan, the third spoke in our snug little wheel. Together, she and Leigh gave me yet another lecture on city etiquette: if you must carry a purse, wear the strap across your chest, don't just loop it over your shoulder; keep your cash separate from your credit cards and ID; keep a spare ten in your shoe so that even if a mugger gets your cash, you can still grab a taxi home; don't give change to panhandlers;

don't talk to strangers; don't *look* at strangers; if somebody starts to follow you, make a scene, don't worry about embarrassing yourself.

"For Pete's sake, I'm not stupid," I said, but my long Midwestern vowels only caused them to collapse into fits of giggles. "Say, 'Jeez!'" they begged me. "Say, 'Goh hohme.' Say, 'Parrk the carr!'"

Now I was laughing, too. What had happened five minutes earlier seemed every bit as unreal, as unrelated to my life, as everything else that happened out there in what we called *the real world,* the world that did not revolve around music, the world we had voluntarily left behind.

As a child, I'd daydreamed about becoming a nun, alternately tantalizing and terrifying myself with the thought that I might have a *vocation,* a calling from God. The Conservatory was very much like what I'd imagined then, a clear-cut, stripped-down little world that simplified your choices, retooled your life around one single, burning thing. We studied music theory, music history, music composition, and conducting. We declared both a major and minor instrument, and prepared recitals in both. We took private lessons, group lessons, master classes, ensemble; we hired ourselves out as ringers in church choirs and local orchestras, gigged at restaurants and coffee shops and bars. Few of us went out on dates, and if we did, we dated other music majors. Some of us held part-time jobs—I ushered at the nearby Morris Mechanic Theater—and if somebody wanted a nonmusic course in math or science or literature, they could always ride a shuttle bus to Johns Hopkins University, with which the Conservatory was affiliated. But mostly, we stayed on campus, in the cloister. Set apart from the distractions of daily life.

Occasionally, a group of us ventured out for breakfast at Sam's, a diner across the street where cockroaches raced up and down the walls. Less frequently, we'd walk down Charles Street to the harbor, where we shopped and watched the street performers. Saturday nights, we might put on our Peabody Conservatory sweatshirts and skulk around outside the Joseph Myerhoff Symphony Hall, alert for someone with an extra ticket: the man whose baby-sitter had canceled and whose wife insisted he come alone; the woman whose friend had the flu; the widow whose husband had died at the beginning of the concert season. When people saw we were Conservatory students, they often gave up their extra ticket for a token amount, if anything at all. "And what instrument do you play?" they'd ask, sweeping us inside, one by one. "And what do you think of tonight's program?"

Afterward, we'd meet in the lobby, then walk back to campus in a large, loose group. The streets always seemed to be shining from rain or, in summer, from the humidity; the sky overhead was a luminous orange. I didn't know anything about light pollution, and for a long time I thought that the Baltimore sky changed color every night for some mysterious reason no one could explain. I loved that sky, that color. I loved the cobblestone streets, the thin sad faces of the row houses, the porches where families sat in hot weather, watching the world pass by. I loved the stink of the buses, the blast of air conditioning that ballooned in front of the banks and public buildings, the drawn, wary faces of men selling jewelry out of slender briefcases.

I loved the Conservatory itself, the sweeping marble stairway that led up toward the teaching studios, the shining black-and-white tiles in the lobby, the extraordinary architecture of the library. I loved the listening lab, the rows of headsets and record players, the tall shelves packed with thousands of recordings. I loved the student body, its range of eccentricities; the particularly robust soprano who'd come to breakfast in a pink, taffeta gown; the drag queens, who arrived for classes transformed by makeup and beautiful shoes; the punk rock trumpet player, who tied shut her broken instrument case with a padlock and chain. The practice rooms stayed open from six in the morning until two A.M. and the collision of so many instruments—an edgy, otherworldly sound—played in the background of every meal, every class, every conversation. It created a kind of living pedal point, a long, held note so constant I almost forgot to hear it, like the church bell at

Saint Mary's back home, ringing at intervals throughout the day. I could go for hours without noticing it, and then, for no particular reason, the sound would come clear: a reminder, a reference point, the tonic key. Home.

Our days began and ended with practice, a routine, a habit, that was very much like prayer. When we weren't actually practicing, we were talking about it: how much we had left to do that day, the room we'd signed up for, the chances of finding extra time in a room nobody had claimed. Practice rooms were chosen every morning though what had come to be known as The Lottery. Promptly at six, a senior RA arrived with the sign-up sheets and a top hat filled with numbered pieces. One by one, we drew the number that determined the order in which we got to reserve the room we'd practice in that day. Drawing a low number meant an acoustically pleasant room with an excellent piano during prime hours. Drawing a high number meant you'd wouldn't get to practice until the wee hours of the morning—unless you were willing to settle for a windowless studio with barely enough room to push back the piano bench, waves of sound thundering from wall to wall like the retort of a howitzer. These were the studios that housed the worst pianos, the crippled and infirm, the geriatric warhorses put out to pasture. Many had fallen victim to composition majors, who'd riddled the strings with paper clips and rubberbands, burned the hammer pads with cigarette lighters, and generally transformed what had been a passable instrument into an atonal misery.

My favorite room, when I could get it, was my piano teacher's studio. It had two good pianos, each with a different action, and tall, west-facing windows that overlooked Charles Square. At night, resting my arms, I'd sit on the window ledge with my feet dangling over the three-story drop, watching the parade of expensive cars trolling up and down Charles Street, circling the Monument, coasting to a stop. Prostitutes stepped forward from the shadows then, silent as deer, and like deer they were long-legged and watchful, gangly in their teetering heels. They bent forward at the waist, pushed back their hair; they seemed to be waiting for something. At last, one would break from the rest to approach the idling car, and now a man's hand would emerge, the glint of a wedding band, a languid elbow resting on the door frame.

My first year at Peabody, I was studying Brahms to my heart's content, working my way through the intermezzi, and there were nights I could almost imagine I was conjuring scenes from the composer's childhood, the seedy Hamburg district where he'd been raised. I loved to imagine him as an adolescent, walking home past the women on the corners, past the bars and beggars, a lonely figure made lonelier still by his talent, his singular, private vision. I loved to imagine his unreturned passion for Clara Schumann, how he'd lived his life alone—without lover or child—until it ended, one year after her death. I believed that the soul of an artist could only be wrought by such personal suffering, could only be redeemed by offering oneself up to Art and Art alone. By fulfilling every sacrifice it demanded. By remaking oneself as an empty vessel to be filled, and filled again.

As a child, I'd read and reread the *Lives of the Saints,* studying the martyrs as if their lives were a map I longed to follow: Saint Martina, who bled milk after the emperor cut off her breasts; Saint Fausta, who endured one thousand nails hammered into her skull; Saint Euphemia, whose limbs were ripped from her body. Now it was the lives of dead composers and living virtuosi I emulated, lingering over their hardships, their sacrifices, their pain. Practice and prayer, music and God, the discipline of the Conservatory and the discipline of the Church—over time, the two had become inextricably intertwined, for the truth was that I needed the first to maintain the second. Music was the purest language I knew, the bridge between what I was supposed to believe and what I knew in my heart to be true. And that truth, too frightening for me to fully acknowledge, was this: I was falling away from the Church. I was *losing my faith.*

Sunday after Sunday, I sat at the back of Saint Ignatius Church, trying my best not to argue with the gospel, with the priest's homily, with the Bible's glorification of violence, bigotry, intolerance. Little things irked me. I had not yet read Bertrand Russell's *Why I Am Not a Christian,* but I, too, couldn't understand why Christ would drive demons out of a man, only to inflict them on a herd of pigs. Why didn't Christ just *kill* the demons, for Pete's sake? I'd grown up with pigs. I *liked* pigs. Weren't they God's creatures, too? Then there was the story of Job, a good man tortured by God, just because He feels the testosterone urge to show off for the devil. And what about Martha's sister, Mary, sitting at Christ's feet? Mary, rubbing those feet with expensive oil and drying them with her hair? Clearly, Christ is enjoying himself like any other red-blooded man, for when Mary's sister, Martha, points out that the oil might have been sold and the proceeds given to the poor, Christ tells her, in effect, to butt out. "The poor will always be with us," he says, "but the son of man comes only once."

Yeah, grumbled my brain, my old *grandfather* would come, if some babe sat between his knees that way, rubbing her hair between his toes.

Then I'd recollect myself. I was thinking about *Christ,* the Son of *God.* God, who could strike me dead if He felt like it. *Shut up, shut up,* I'd tell my brain, and when it rebelled, I flooded it with Hail Marys. I pinched my thigh beneath my Sunday skirt. I tried to prepare myself to take Communion, the actual body and blood of Christ, into the temple of the Holy Ghost that was my body.

So you're a cannibal, is that it? jeered my brain.

It was hopeless. I fled the church in despair, returned to the practice rooms.

It was words, I finally decided, that were at the root of my trouble. How could you worship something as infinite as God with something as finite as language? No wonder I was tormented by doubts, contradictions, oxymorons that couldn't be reconciled. Faith had to rise above all that while words, born of reason, pulled you down into the muck, rubbed your face in your own human quirks and questionings. I hated words, their gradations and shadings, the way a thing could be argued one way, slanted another, depending on who was using it. I'd left my required freshman comp course with a gentlewoman's C, delighted by the thought that I'd never again have to analyze another poem, or story, or essay.

So then why couldn't I stop analyzing my faith?

I made an appointment with the sweet old priest at Saint Ignatius, and together, we arrived at this analogy. The world was very much like a complicated piece of music. When you first saw the score, you couldn't make sense of anything right away. It seemed chaotic, random, out of control. But if you broke everything down, page by page, stanza by stanza, over time you came to understand what sounds went where and why. You saw that the notes were a kind of path leading to a place you'd never seen before, and yet, had always been there, waiting for you to notice. The fault had been in the limitation of the beholder, not the breadth and scope of the view. That's why it was important to trust God, who had a better view of things, a more complete picture, than you alone ever could.

I thanked the old priest gratefully. I wanted so desperately to believe what he was saying—for the sake of my soul, but also for the sake of my physical self. I wanted to believe that the same truth could apply to what was happening to me. My arms were growing more and more painful, and yet I forced myself to the practice rooms, where I put in four and five hours of practice each day. If it were God's will for me to hurt this way, I would have to accept it as part of His plan. This, like all things, was happening for a reason, and all these reasons were born like seeds within the infinite mind of God.

The thought of ceasing to believe in such logic, of stepping away from it, of embracing my life as an open-ended mystery left me feeling as if I was falling, falling, like one of those dreams in which you wake up just before you land. How could you live in the world if you didn't believe in cause and effect, in a greater pattern and purpose? If you didn't trust that the trials you faced were designed for you specifically by a loving and all-knowing God? This idea got complicated whenever I thought about things like droughts and plagues and genocide, so, well, I simply didn't think about those things. No, I believed in my own self-importance; I believed in the sparrow's fall. If I tripped walking out of music theory, there must be a reason beyond my own embarrassment: a lesson to be learned, a purposeful delay that would keep me from arriving in the next moment ahead of schedule. I thanked God for allowing me to trip. I put myself fully into His hands. Everything was a sign of his favor or, at least, His recognition, and if I wasn't able to interpret these signs, the fault could be only my own.

"Can I ask you something?" Susan said one day as we came back from the showers. "Why do you keep a penny pinned to your underwear?"

A penny? Could she mean my old Saint Benedict medal, which I still wore, hanging it from a little gold pin? Each pair of underwear I owned had a series of pinprick holes around the waistband; when I showered, I held the medal in my mouth, so that I wouldn't be parted from it even for a moment. I tried to explain about Saint Benedict, about the vow I'd taken when I was a child, about protection from Satan. I tried, and then I stopped. It all sounded ridiculous. It *was* ridiculous and, yet, I couldn't let it go.

"I wear it," I told her honestly, fighting tears, "because I am afraid to take it off."

Susan nodded kindly, diplomatically. She was, by her own definition, 'culturally Jewish.' "You want me to sit with you while you try?"

We went to her room, still in our robes, and sat down on her bed. I unpinned my Saint Benedict medal and handed it to her. By now I was sobbing. I knew the devil was going to get me. I knew my arms were hurting as punishment for my doubts. I also knew that such thoughts were absolute nonsense. At last, I understood the Holy Trinity: three states of mind in one.

"Do you want it back?" Susan asked, but I shook my head. What I wanted was the smug security of my childhood faith, everything divided into rules and rows laid out as clearly as a cornfield. *Ask and ye shall receive. Faith the size of a mustard seed grain.* What I wanted was to return to the deep sleep of that faith. What I wanted was my arms to feel better.

Even in the fall of my sophomore year, when I had to start wearing night splints, I did not cut back on my practicing. Conservatory students thought of themselves as athletes; no pain, no gain. I was careful to remove the splints before I left my room, so nobody would find out. Leigh knew about them, of course, the way she knew I'd been going to a sports medicine specialist at Johns Hopkins for ultrasound therapy and shots of cortisone. Susan knew about the splints, too, but nobody else did—not even my piano teacher. An actual injury was serious, but rumors of an injury could be equally damaging. When chamber music groups were assembled, when nominations for awards were announced, when lists declared which of us were eligible for scholarships and competitions, the names of the injured—those who were inconsistent, unreliable—were conspicuously absent.

Yet, injuries were commonplace, particularly among pianists, particularly among female pianists. A girl one floor down from me fractured her arm landing a Beethoven chord. Another suffered permanent nerve damage in her right fourth finger. Nearly everyone, regardless of their instrument, went to the practice rooms armed with a variety of compresses, wraps and Ace bandages, sports creams, and anti-inflammatories. The air reeked of Tiger Balm and Ben-Gay and Aspercreme. In the dorms, there was always someone lying on a heating pad. We scheduled appointments for vitamin shots and physical therapy and Swedish massage, and when these treatments failed, we caught the train to D.C. where there was an acupuncturist—his telephone number was passed hand to hand—who gave discounts to Conservatory students. And if Dr. Xu couldn't help you, well, then you gritted your teeth and *played through*. Now and then, somebody else would pack up their dorm room and head back home, ostensibly to return after a semester of "rest," which meant we would never see them again. We mourned them, of course, but recovered soon enough to squabble over the gigs they'd abandoned, the seats they'd vacated in the various ensembles. There was always a sense that the people who left were the ones who hadn't *wanted it enough,* the ones who hadn't been *hungry. We,* the survivors, were the hungry ones. We were eager to be tested, to prove ourselves. We were in our teens and early twenties, the age when you believe you control your own life like a beautiful kite on the end of a string.

My hero that fall was one of the master instructors, an internationally renowned pianist who'd been unable to perform for a decade until, thanks to est and lecithin, the tendinitis in his hands began to heal. A comeback performance had already been scheduled with the Baltimore Symphony Orchestra for the spring. It was to be a gala event, and everybody talked about the way a lesser man would have given up, packed in the towel, settled into an honorable teaching career. Whenever the burning in my forearms and wrists forced me to pause during a lesson, my own instructor reminded me of the master instructor's difficulties—and his upcoming triumph.

"It takes heart," my instructor would say, spraying my outstretched arms with a topical analgesic she ordered from Germany. It came in a slender, silver can, and it felt like ice when it hit your skin. She kept a second can by the door so you could blast yourself when you first came in. "Do you have heart? Because if you don't, get the hell off the Good Ship Lollipop."

She had two stock lectures she administered to students in her studio, reinoculating us throughout the semester. The first, and most frequent, was *Never End Up a Teacher.* The second was *Never Marry for Love.* "Marry for love," she'd say, "and you'll spend your life raising puppies."

They didn't make women like that in Wisconsin. I adored her. If she'd told me to practice with thumbtacks pushed into my fingertips, I'd probably have obeyed.

She was somewhere in her thirties and dramatically beautiful, and when I looked at the man she'd married—a bulbous old fool of a violinist who spent most of his energy attempting to seduce his undergraduates—it was clear she was in no danger of falling victim to anybody's charms. Her career as a performer had come to an end because of chronic back pain; she often walked with a cane. On particularly bad days, she stood through the lesson. On worse days still, she paced, her breath coming in hard little puffs. I left the studio feeling as if my own pain was nothing but an excuse, a symptom of my own lack of focus. I resolved to work harder. I ate lecithin like gumdrops. I got another round of cortisone shots, swallowed aspirin until my ears rang, renewed my prescriptions for anti-inflammatories and then lied to the doctor about the side effects: abdominal pain, diarrhea, weight loss. I even visited the acupuncturist, but by the end of my third semester, I couldn't shampoo my hair properly because I couldn't keep my arms raised above my head that long. Instead, I slapped the shampoo on my head, then stood directly under the shower stream, hoping the force of the water would drill the soap into my hair.

Fortunately, I could keep my arms at waist level while I was playing the piano, but other problems were cropping up: holding a pencil to take notes, gripping a knife to cut meat, lowering something down from my high closet shelf. Trying to run scales, I slurred notes hopelessly, and there were times my hands grew so numb I had to look to see where they were. When I spoke to my parents on the phone, the receiver kept slipping out of my grasp.

"Fine, everything's fine," I said. "Just dropped the phone."

And then there were the problems I was having with, well, my legs. Who had ever heard of such a thing? My legs weren't nearly as bad as my arms, but if I walked too far too fast, they'd start to burn, and when I jogged, it took several days to recover. Pain up and down my shins, along the insides of my legs from ankle to knee, sometimes across the top of my feet, particularly my right foot. Sometimes, this foot didn't quite want to pull up after I'd take a step, and this mystified and embarrassed me.

Now I was truly frightened. Was I psychosomatically ill? I made another appointment with the sports medicine specialist I'd been seeing at Johns Hopkins. He injected my wrists and elbows with more cortisone and had me fitted with new wrist braces I was supposed to wear while I was practicing, writing, cutting up food. Then he sent me to another specialist, a neurologist, who had me walk around the exam room so that he could *evaluate my gait.* He asked me to close my eyes and touch my nose. He pricked my feet with pins and asked if it felt dull or sharp.

"Your right foot gets tired?" he said. He thought about it for a moment. "Which foot do you use to work the pedals on the piano?"

"The right, mostly," I said.

"Try using your left foot instead."

I felt stupid for bringing it up.

In December 1983, I headed home to Wisconsin for winter break. There, for the next three weeks, I took my health seriously. I forced myself to take a break from the piano—no cheating, no short sessions, nothing. I wore my wrist braces every day. I washed down the anti-inflammatories with milkshakes and big, starchy meals, trying to console my stomach. Mornings, I slept late; afternoons, I visited relatives; nights, I watched videos with friends. I spent a week out at Grandma Krier's farm, sleeping beside her in the old double bed just as I had when I was younger. She had sent a check to Rome in November, after my mother had first told her about the problems I was having.

Any day now, she assured me, a Mass would be said for my intentions. Any day now, I should be feeling better.

And by the end of my vacation, I could report, truthfully, that I did feel much better than I had. I was sleeping through the night again; my arms and legs no longer woke me with their buzz and burn. I could walk all the way from her house to Great Uncle Joe and Aunt Eleanor's, a quarter mile down the road, and sit in their living room quite comfortably, admiring their Christmas tree.

"Take it easy," my mother pleaded with me as she drove me back to the airport. I promised I would, and I kept that promise. Back in Baltimore, I took the bus to my part-time job at the theater. I practiced no more than two hours a day. But within a few weeks, all my symptoms had returned. I couldn't keep up with my piano lesson preps, and in March, I withdrew from ensemble. I relied on the braces more and more, not only at the piano, but taking notes, raising and lowering my cereal spoon, anything that required repetitive motion. By now, my injuries were common knowledge, impossible to conceal, and when midsemester grades came due, my teacher told me that the time had come to stop making excuses.

"I understand," I said, forcing myself to look unconcerned. We'd just spent yet another lesson on music theory, because I hadn't been able to prepare that week's assignment.

"No, you don't," she said. "I'm giving the A you would

have had, if it weren't for all this." She waved her hands at my braces.

"Thank you," I said.

"*Don't* thank me," she said. "*Listen* to me. If this doesn't resolve itself soon, you'll need to rethink your major." She gave me a hard, keen look that wasn't without sympathy. "There's a good music therapy program at Hopkins," she said. "I had a student several years back who transferred, graduated on schedule, got a job working at a clinic somewhere. A good job. Something with autistic children. I could make a few calls."

It had been a long time since she'd talked to me about the master instructor, held up his difficulties as an example, reminded me that all it took was heart—an omission that seemed particularly telling, for his comeback performance was only a week away. You couldn't open up the local paper without seeing something about it. There were posters up on every bulletin board. There'd been an interview on public radio. Did she think I'd lost my drive? Did she think I wanted to settle down and raise puppies? I couldn't believe that she, of all people, was suggesting I become a teacher.

"That will not be necessary," I said. I spoke as firmly as I could. "I'm going to get better."

"Of course you're going to get better," she snapped. "But when? Because you don't have two, three, five years to wait. If you're going to have a career, things need to happen for you now. You've already lost a semester, and frankly, I don't foresee any improvement."

I left the studio furious, determined to show my teacher she was wrong. Who was to say I wouldn't recover? Who was to say this wouldn't be just one of many marvelous anecdotes I'd tell some day, after I became successful, after I'd demonstrated the power of positive thinking? The master instructor's public radio interview had been filled with such marvelous anecdotes. He was practicing hard these days, getting ready; I sometimes sat outside his practice room door to listen. I figured that if I couldn't practice myself, the next best thing was hearing somebody else at work, following along with the score. I got permission to sit in on friends' lessons. I spent hours in the listening lab, memorizing concertos and symphonies.

Susan offered to teach me how to hypnotize myself. Her father, a psychiatrist, had taught her how to do it, and she hypnotized herself before performances so that she wouldn't feel nervous. First thing in the morning and last thing at night, I sat with my eyes rolled back in my head, suggesting affirmations to my subconscious. *My wrists feel warm and good. My hands are powerful and strong.*

On the night of the master instructor's comeback performance, I walked to the symphony hall alone. Months earlier, I'd splurged on a single orchestra seat, and now I kept my hand in my pocket so I could feel the ticket between my fingers. For once, I wouldn't be scrounging for a ticket, worrying about whether or not I'd get in and where, if I did, I would sit. It was a warm April night, and I wore only my Peabody sweatshirt over a loose, flowing skirt, cotton tights, and lace-up boots, a dozen cloth bracelets on my wrists. My hair had grown long and, since leaving home, I'd learned to wear it straight. Tonight, I'd pulled it back with a ribbon. I wore earrings and perfume. I'd fussed in a way that I almost never fussed, and I'd left early so I could be there to watch the concert hall fill up.

All day, my mouth had been dry, the way it always got before my own performances. In a sense, this was my own performance; at least, this is what I had come to believe. For if everything went well, I would understand that my own pain had been but a momentary setback, something that would pass. I had prayed over this and fasted over this and now I believed it with all my heart. I wasn't expecting a miracle—no. Just a wing-brush of God's compassion, an easing of this terrible uncertainty I felt I could no longer bear. Tonight, I would finally have an answer to the question I'd been asking for months: do I still have a future in music? And so I was going to the concert. I would listen with an open heart. I would drink the notes into my aching arms like medicine.

"If a child asks his father for bread," I reminded myself, "will he hand him a scorpion?"

I arrived just as the doors were opening. The crowd pressed forward, catching me with it, sweeping me inside on a wave of bow ties and black dresses and pearls. By the time I found my seat, the orchestra was already half full, and when I turned around, I saw the crowds surging into the balconies. Good concerts give you chills; great concerts give you chills before they even begin. It was clear that this was going to be one of the greats, a night to remember. When the lights came down and the master instructor stepped onto the stage, a collective *ah!* rose from the audience, a single exhalation of joy. The applause didn't build; it simply arrived like a good, hard rain, continued as if it could go on all night. A few people shouted *Bravo!* but the master instructor lifted his hands a little—*please, please,* he seemed to be saying—and then seated himself at the piano, where he waited for the crowd to settle down. Still, the applause drummed the air. The conductor grinned like a schoolboy. People all around me, strangers, were exchanging nods and smiles. *See,* we all were saying to each other, *there he is, he's back.* I reminded myself of the old priest's analogy. Even I could see, now, that all those years of misery had had their purpose Without them a moment this sweet, this grand, could never have existed.

At last, the conductor raised his baton. We all leaned forward. The concerto began. But ten minutes into the first movement, the clean lines of the master instructor's melodies started to blur. People behind me murmured uneasily; heads moved side to side. The conductor gradually slowed the tempo, but by the time the master instructor had arrived at the cadenza, I could see very clearly how his right hand was refusing to articulate, how the fourth and fifth fingers kept knuckling under. Still, he lumbered along, a Herculean effort, until he reached the bitter end only slightly behind the orchestra. His face was slick with sweat as he rose, clutching his right hand with his left, as if to wring out the pain. The applause sounded different than it had before. It rose into shrillness and kept on rising, an unpleasant, pitying sound. Again and again, the master instructor bowed—helplessly, automatically, unable to creep away—and I saw in his rigid expression something of my own face, my own determination, my own belief that, with enough will, enough faith, anything was possible. Here, standing before me, was a ghost of the best future I might hope for, an endless cycle of hope and despair, false starts, comebacks that were never fully realized. And even that, I knew, was far more than would be my portion. The master instructor had been trained by other master instructors since his childhood; he'd developed his injuries at the height of a young, but brilliant, career. My own career had barely begun and, to be fair, I had never been any kind of genius. I was yet another talented student, one of hundreds, full of heart.

I stood up and began climbing over people's knees, desperate to escape. Outside, the air had cooled; the streets were steaming, surreal. I walked like somebody in a dream, not heading anywhere in particular. Men called to me, a nagging fugue that waxed and waned: *Hey baby, hey sweetheart, nice legs, like to see what's between 'em.* For the past two years, day or night, alone or with other women, I had not once stepped out from behind the Conservatory walls and not heard that same ugly music, a variation on the same theme I'd heard from the wrestlers in high school. An embellishment of what I saw on TV, in movies, in slick magazines. The flip side of the Church's focus on female virginity, chastity, purity. In the past, I'd always assured myself that I was above *all* such imagery. Church or street, Madonna or whore, I was, after all, an artist. It had nothing to do with me.

Except that it did. Or at least, from now on, it would.

Hey baby, hey sweetheart. Show us your tits.

Who would I be without the piano? Legs and arms, a body, a face—all of it without meaning beyond the dull physical facts? *Your body is God's temple* floated into my head, a reflex like a sob, but the words meant nothing. They rattled inside my emptiness like stones dropped into a can. I would have to stop playing the piano, I understood that now. I would leave the Conservatory at the end of the school year. As for the Catholic Church, I realized I'd left that long ago; I'd merely been clinging to the shreds out of fear, obligation, habit. *Let it go,* I told myself and, amazingly, I did. The whole anxiety-ridden knot of it floated up out of my hands and into the sky, carrying my music along with it.

For the first time in my life, there was nothing but silence in my head. No thoughts of music. No thoughts of God. How would I ever fill such a space? Who would I become? I was falling through the streets of Baltimore, falling through the surface of the earth. Only this time I wasn't dreaming, I wasn't sleeping, I was waking up and, try as I might, I would never go back to sleep again. Even my name, *Ann, Ann Manette,* tasted unfamiliar in my mouth.

A man had been trailing me in his car; now he rolled down his window, offered me fifty bucks to get in. Sixty dollars. Seventy-five. "That would pay for a whole lot of music books," he said, and I spun around to look at him before I remembered I was wearing my Peabody sweatshirt.

"Made you look," the man said, laughing. He was white, middle-aged, handsome. He wore a light coat open over his business suit and tie. A fat gold wedding band. He could have been my father. He could have been someone who cared about me. He was somebody's husband, somebody's child, and I wanted to get in his car, to sit beside him, to tell him everything. He must have seen that in my face and misunderstood.

"One hundred dollars," he said. "C'mon, that's more than you're worth."

I believed him. I burst into tears, startling us both.

"Hey," he began, but I was already running, and I ran until I got to Charles Street, where it was crowded and bright and safe. I went into a coffee bar where I tried to collect myself, while the waiters—beautiful and muscled and gay—brought me water and tissues, a glass of wine, rubbed my shoulders and called me *honey* and promised to seriously mess up whoever it was who had hurt me.

But no, I wasn't hurt. No, there wasn't anything anybody could do. When no one was looking, I left money on the table and hurried outside onto Charles Street. Then I headed back toward the Conservatory, legs aching from the running I'd done, swinging my right foot a little to keep from tripping on the toe.

Part Three

Nine

P*oint of view* is the vantage point from which the world is observed, the story is told. If that vantage point changes, the point of view *shifts,* and the story reshapes itself to accommodate the new perspective. One landscape is lost; another is gained. The distance between is called *vision.*

I got my first power wheelchair in May 1987, a few months before my twenty-third birthday, eighteen months after I'd first come home from Maine for what I'd thought would be a few weeks of medical leave. It was an Everest & Jennings, a monster of a thing: black seat, black wheelie-bars, black swing-away legs with shiny chrome footrests that stuck out in front of it like bared teeth. I'd ordered it that way. No colors, no racing stripes. None of the chirpy, cheery accessories the dealer promised would make me *approachable.*

"Nice Death Star," my brother said dryly, the first time he saw it.

We navigate our lives by the random light of symbols, concrete objects that shimmer with meaning—accurate or imagined. When I was twenty-two, a power chair stood for my greatest fear: dependence, weakness, failure. As the dealer demonstrated the joystick, the speed control, the battery charger, I felt as if I were preparing to renounce my citizenship, to cross some unimaginable border into a flat, colorless country where I'd live out my life in exile from everything that had made me who I was. Never mind that without it, I was living with my parents in a state of isolation, dragging myself between the bedroom and the bathroom, with an occasional detour to the living room couch for a mind-numbing dose of television. It could always be worse, I'd told myself. It's not like I'm in a wheelchair or something. The folding wheelchair we'd rented from the drugstore didn't count; it was, after all, just temporary. It was just something I sat in to, you know, get places.

"Ready for a test drive?" the dealer asked. He patted the seat as if it were a tricycle and I was a shy kindergartner. "All aboard!"

My mother looked at him sharply, then glanced at me. The word *asshole* appeared in my mind, and I knew she'd put it there. Earlier, when she'd pushed me into the dealership, he'd greeted us by asking her, "So! Is this the new quad?" Through the plate glass window, I could see out into the parking lot where my father was pacing around and around my new and newly customized Ford van. We all watched as he stopped at the control panel that operated the wheelchair lift, bent to insert the key. The lift went up, came down, went up again. Our insurance was covering the power chair, but my parents had paid for the van and its modifications out of pocket. There was no other way to transport the chair. It did not fold. It was too heavy to lift.

My parents were kind enough to pretend I was going to be able to pay them back soon.

I hauled myself out of the push chair, took the two steps to the E & J, and sank into the seat.

"Hey, you stand up pretty good!" the dealer crowed. "How does that feel? Should we lengthen the legs a little?"

"They're fine," I said, mortified.

"Terrific." He reached across my lap to turn down the speed control. "Take a spin around the room," he said. "Let's see how you do."

I turned the speed control back up.

"A daredevil!" he said. Then, turning to my mother: "They're all that way. Put 'em in a chair, and the next thing you know, they're zipping up and down the sidewalks like race car drivers."

Get me away from this guy, I thought, and I waited for my mother to complete my thought by pulling me back, turning me around. Our lives had become so intimate, so closely intertwined, that we often read each other's thoughts, said the same thing at the same time. My mother could usually anticipate where I wanted to go, how fast I wanted to get there, when I wanted to stop. Now, however, she did nothing, merely stepped back a little. That was when it hit me: I could move independently. I could decide which way I wanted to go without communicating this to anybody. Even using crutches had meant a certain amount of team effort: I couldn't carry anything; I couldn't open doors; I needed somebody to run ahead and make sure there would be a place to sit down. At home, I knew how many steps I'd need to get myself through the day, and these steps were budgeted, rationed, tallied, for I didn't have any to spare. In new situations, my mother ran ahead like a military scout, returned with the information we needed to plan my advance. *There are two steps up if we go in this way,* she'd say, *but there's a radiator you can perch on as soon as you get to the top; the other way is longer, but there aren't any steps, and there's a bathroom on the way.* We always kept an eye out for bathrooms. If we saw one I could get to, I used it whether I needed to or not. You never knew how long it would be until the next one came along.

The power chair was about to change all that.

I touched the joystick, and the chair lurched forward, surprising me. I had tried a power chair in Rochester, under the supervision of a physical therapist, but that had been a battered old granddaddy of a chair, with a headrest like a vise grip, and fuzzy sheepskin covers on the footrests. Its top speed had been a careful walking pace. To turn a corner, you had to swing wide.

"Let me turn down the speed—" the dealer began, but as he reached toward me, I backed up, clattering into a row of walkers. He leapt to catch them, and I spun around in place, veered around my mother, and headed down the main aisle of the store. When the automatic doors opened, I continued outside. On a whim. On an *impulse.*

It was the first spontaneous thing I'd done in nearly two years.

Outside, it was one of those perfect spring days when the Midwestern sky turns impossibly blue. I circled the van and found my father on the other side, scratching at something on the paint. When he straightened up, I saw myself—my new self, sitting in the power chair—reflected back in the mirrored lenses of his sunglasses. I realized I was seeing what, from now on, other people would see, with all its associations. The image my father was seeing for the first time. The reality of my illness, its impact on our lives.

"Sweetie," he said. His voice was shaking. He ducked his head, then turned away so I could not see his face.

I had thought it would be difficult: going back to college in a wheelchair. Passing through narrow doors, locating ramps and elevators, navigating the crowded cafeteria and the dim aisles of the library. Attending my classes without taking notes; having exams administered orally. Making friends and falling in love. Graduating. Moving on.

It was, in these ways, remarkably easy. Life is not a thriller, a hyped-up movie-of-the-week. Its plot isn't crafted. Its revelations are often retrospective and mild. If you weep, if you rage, if you slump down in defeat, there is no one to see you do it, and so—like a child's tantrum—the inclination passes. You can't help noticing that on days you do not weep, you look better in the mirror, and you manage to accomplish more. You relearn, without drama or sentimentality, how to do the things you need to do. You learn to accept help graciously when something you need to do cannot be done. Eventually, a few weedy tendrils of curiosity poke through the dormant soil, and though you yank them up at first, refusing to be consoled, you are aware, even as you do so, of your own melodrama. When more appear, you let them grow. Soon you even plant a few seeds. Suddenly, you are busy with another thriving garden. Things that have been lost to you make room for others you'd never have planted, were you not motivated to consider other options. Had you not been forced to look around, make different choices for yourself.

A year or so after I started using the power chair, I dreamed that I lived in a two-story house, and that the upper story was filled with all my belongings. In my dream, I was standing at the foot of the stairs, my wheelchair beside me, and I was overwhelmed with sadness because I knew that I couldn't get back up the stairs to retrieve my things. After a while, I noticed that the downstairs wasn't empty, as I'd first thought, but nicely furnished. My belongings were everywhere, scattered between other things, many of which I didn't recognize. But when I looked at them more closely, I realized they were mine after all.

I awoke from the dream feeling as if something had eased. So many of us can divide our lives into episodes: before and after. Before the accident, the heart attack, the cancer. After the war, the divorce, the child's death. The abyss opens beneath our feet, and we leap it, *not* because we are particularly brave, but simply because we must. We land in a whole new country. We put on its clothing, learn its customs, begin again. And yet, the events of our lives still form a single continuum. The things we have experienced go on to shape the things we will experience, a year from now, ten years from now, in ways we can't possibly imagine.

This is what I mean when I say it has been easy. It is only in ways I could not have imagined that it hasn't been easy at all.

Today, it's the man on the street corner, whose eye I have accidentally met. I'm late for a meeting, willing the red light to turn green, so when he says, *I have a lot of respect for someone like you,* the blank look I give him—is genuine.

Someone *like me?*

After the meeting, I duck into a market for groceries, buy flowers from a vendor. The meeting has gone well, and now my head is full of a proposal I must write in collaboration with a friend. But I manage to remember the letter in my purse, a letter I've been carrying around for days, a letter that should have gone out a week ago. I swing back to the post office, get in line, and I'm smoothing the worst of the wrinkles from the envelope when the woman in front of me turns around. *You're seem awfully young to be in one of those things,* she says, mournfully. *Is it permanent?*

We are at the post office. We are waiting in line for stamps. My health, my body, is the furthest thing from my mind, and so it takes me a moment before I hear, another moment still before I understand. Because the woman pities me, she believes I am to be pitied. Because my disability looms large in her mind, she assumes it's the only thing *I'm* thinking of. To her, to the man on the street corner, to the strangers and first-time acquaintances who make these remarks most frequently, I'm merely a body on a set of wheels. A fact without a context.

Women tend to pitch their voices high, as if speaking to a toddler on a tricycle. *Wow, you're really GOOD with that thing! How fast can you go?* Men are more likely to use falsely hearty tones, making wheelchair "jokes," the same ones, over and over. *Hey, wanna race? You should get a snowplow for that thing. Do you take hitchhikers?* Perhaps, the most bewildering remarks are variations on this theme: *You've got it easy—the rest of us have to walk* or *I'm going have to get one of those things for myself.* For it's evident such people don't want one of "these things" for themselves; on the contrary, it's clear they see nothing about me to envy and everything to fear. Obviously, I'm not speedy. Obviously, most people can walk faster, certainly run faster, without much effort.

The summer I first got my E & J, I'd literally gape in amazement—in the grocery store, at the bank, in the student union—each time somebody leapt forward like a bugaboo to cry, *Look out, I'll give you a speeding ticket! Hey, you got a license for that thing?* Perhaps it's me, I thought. Perhaps I'm doing something wrong. It was kind of like hazing, I figured, something that would fade once I got more experience in the chair, once I learned to—but what was it I could learn? Five years later, when I replaced my wheelchair with a three-wheeled scooter, the comments became even more frequent. In recent years, I have taught at universities and summer writers' conferences where the simple act of crossing a room has triggered, day after day, week and week, the same round of uneasy remarks: *Don't run me over! Can I have a ride?*

There are times when my gratitude for a simple *Hi,* for a *How'd your class go?* or *What did you do today?* has made me want to weep. When I refuse—unfairly, I know—to make eye contact with anyone I don't know well, I brace myself against the comments, the inevitable questions: *So how come you use that thing? What's the matter with you?* I turn my speed control to high. I move through the crowd as fast as I can.

One of the last times I saw my Grandma Ansay, I convinced her to take a short walk with me. It was the summer after my first year at Peabody. I was home for a visit, restless, counting the days until I could head back east, and I didn't think I could bear to spend the entire afternoon inside that stifling house. "Just to the end of the block," I told her. "You can hold on to my arm."

"Oh, oh," my grandmother sighed.

I went to the window and pulled back the curtain. The day was as vibrant, as bright, as the living room was airless and dark. "Look," I told my grandmother, who was cowering back, one hand raised in a kind of Dracula pose. "It's gorgeous out there. The nicest day of the year."

"Oh, say," my grandmother said, but after a series of fretful sounds, sniffs, and fragmented words, she surprised me by going to the front hall closet and fishing out her long, wool coat. I helped her into it, pretending not to notice how elaborately she winced while poking her arms through the sleeves. In the process, she dropped her cane.

"No, no," she wailed, as it hit the linoleum floor with a *crack.*

"It's OK, Grandma," I said, "I'll get it, don't worry about it."

"No," she said again, but more calmly, and she took the initiative to reach into her pocket, draw out a flowery scarf and tie it tightly beneath her chin. I was in shorts and a T-shirt, flip-flops. I handed her the cane and, together, we headed out the door.

My grandmother had been a beauty in her youth, and even now, despite the stroke, depression, and inactivity, her skin was luminous, her cheekbones perfectly sculpted, and when she raised her head you saw how very tall she was, how queenly. It was a Saturday morning and the neighborhood was quiet: rectangular ranch houses quartered on rectangular lots, two-car driveways facing the street, neatly trimmed and fertilized lawns so green that they seemed unreal. A single car idled somewhere up the street. A lone child ran through a sprinkler. The scrape of my grandmother's orthopedic shoes was like the cry of an unfamiliar bird: a questioning rasp, then a pause, another rasp. We didn't talk as we walked, because all of her concentration was focused on the left side of her body, lifting her knee, dropping her foot on the sidewalk, then taking a step with her good leg and dragging the left one after it. She was breathing hard. From time to time we stopped so she could rest. But for once, she wasn't complaining. She wasn't moaning, drawing attention to herself. She had made up her mind to walk to the corner, and we were nearly there when one of her neighbors, a man in his fifties, came out of his house. For a moment, he stood on his porch, watching our progress. Then:

"Hey, there, young lady!" he called.

I'd assumed he was talking to me. "Yes, sir?"

The man stepped off his porch and crossed the lawn to the sidewalk. "I meant the *young* lady," he said, speaking in a falsely hearty voice. "Margaret, it's so good to see you out for a change!"

My grandmother made a choked, little sound.

"And who is this?" he asked, indicating me. "Must be your older sister, am I right?"

I was seventeen and my grandmother was in her eighties. This time, my grandmother didn't attempt to respond.

"This is my *grandmother,*" I told the man with great dignity.

The man laughed as if I'd told a good joke. "Well, I won't

hold you girls up," he said. "Stay out of trouble now, Margaret."

He winked at my grandmother, the way you might wink at a child, before heading back into the house.

My grandmother had stopped walking; she leaned heavily on my arm. We stood in the middle of the sidewalk, and the very air around us seemed to glitter with her rage and humiliation. "It's OK," I kept saying, but it wasn't OK, and when at last she turned back toward the house, I did not protest.

The year I got my power chair, I often recalled that day; even now, when people say the things they say, I think about my grandmother. How ironic that I've finally come to understand her, to empathize, now that it's too late. Like my grandmother, I find it hard to go out, to enter unfamiliar situations. I cherish my family, my small circle of friends, but I have to force myself to keep up with acquaintances, develop new relationships. *Hey, recluse, pick up the phone!* begins the latest string of unreturned messages on my answering machine. Then I remember my grandmother's house, the drawn curtains, the stale air. I force myself to return a few calls. I order myself outside.

Today, it's a beautiful autumn day. I put on sunglasses, hook the dog to my scooter, and take him for a walk in the park. He's a few paces behind me, angling to snag something disgusting off the sidewalk, when I hear a woman loudly pointing me out to her children.

See that lady? she says. *That lady is blind.*

I begin to laugh, I can't help myself. I laugh until I cry.

I once heard a radio interview with a writer who'd lost everything in a house fire. The young, eager interviewer suggested that, perhaps, the event could be construed as a lucky one, for despite the initial tragedy, the writer had been left with the ability to start his life fresh, clean. There was a shocked silence before the writer replied, and though I don't remember exactly what he said, I remember how his voice shook as he tried, unsuccessfully, to conceal his anger and dismay. Didn't the interviewer understand that everything the writer had lost, even now, remained incomprehensible? Manuscripts and correspondence, photographs and antiques, things that had been in his family for generations, things that could never be replaced. Evidence of his passions, the physical path of his comings and goings, all that had documented his passage through the world—how could the interviewer suggest such a loss could be anything like *lucky?*

There was a brief silence on the air. And I remembered a time when I was newly disabled, in constant and grueling pain. A slight acquaintance—who knows why?—started nattering on about how I should consider myself lucky to have fallen ill, to be in a wheelchair, to have such a unique perspective on the world. I stared at my lap, too angry to speak, waiting for her to finish and walk away on her two strong legs, but no, she kept at it, kept digging herself in deeper, until at last something came apart inside my head and I snapped—cruelly, yes, unforgivably—"Well, then I hope something terrible happens to you, so you'll have all the same opportunities."

Loss is loss; grief is grief. Even now, I understand the writer's longing for those photographs, how he must look back from time to time and wish he'd paid attention, studied them more closely. And what if he'd consigned them to a safe deposit box, the way he'd always meant to do? What if the fire had stopped with the kitchen, a little smoke damage, scorched curtains, nothing more? Who among us can honestly say that such thoughts never buzz against the screens, try as we will to chase them all out?

Yet I do understand, in theory, what the interviewer meant, what the acquaintance was trying to say. As a child, I was told that *when God closes a door, He opens a window.* As an adult, taking responsibility not only for my weaknesses and faults but for my strengths and capabilities, I see that *every* experience—positive, negative, and in between—contains multiple windows, large and small, if we make up our minds to find them. Still, there are times when the force of the door leaves us damaged beyond reason. When, like birds, we lie stunned for a minute, for an hour, and it isn't clear to anyone whether we'll ever come to, fly away.

Ten

Writing fiction began for me as a side effect of illness, a way to live beyond my body when it became clear that this new, altered body would be mine to keep. A way to fill the hours that had once been occupied by music. A way to achieve the kind of closure that, once, I'd found through prayer. Years later, a writer I admire would tell me of awakening in the hospital after a car wreck at the age of eight, and thinking, with absolute clarity: "Now I can be anything, and I want to be a writer."

On January 1, 1988, I made a New Year's resolution to write for two hours, three times a week. Even now, twelve years later, I cannot explain why I made this particular resolution and not another—to become a painter, say, or to compose an opera. I might have taken up singing. I might have found religion again, joined another church. I might have done any number of things that would have been more, as I would say now, *in character.* My adult fiction reading had been limited to grocery store romances, the kind with half-corseted breasts peeping through the cover. The only sustained writing I'd done, aside from college papers, were the poems I'd scrawled whenever I fancied myself miserable or in love. The latter, which I'd collected in a cloth-covered notebook, had mysteriously disappeared during my first semester at the University of Maine. Choice excerpts had resurfaced, however, on bulletin boards across campus, and for a while guys I didn't know kept calling to ask if I wanted to come over and see their rooms. This had left me feeling somewhat uneasy about poetry. Occasionally, I'd had a vague idea about starting a novel, but I figured that writing—like falling in love, or saving money, or working crossword puzzles—was something I could always do later in life, when I got older and less active, when I needed something I could do sitting down.

On New Year's Eve, 1987, at the age of twenty-three, it occurred to me that this was exactly my situation.

During the eighteen months I'd been on medical leave, I'd made countless similar resolutions. I'd planned the various trips I'd take as soon as I got well—to the Australian outback, to the Galápagos Islands, to Anchorage, Alaska. I completed a correspondence course on beekeeping, dreamed of my own hives on a little plot of land in Maine. I researched llamas and ostriches and beefalo, considered starting a farm, or a bed-and-breakfast, or both. From time to time, I'd scrap all these ideas in favor of living on a sailboat. I wrote away for information on boat-building schools and sailing academies; I studied the Chapman guide to seamanship, savoring words like *ketch* and *yawl*. But in each of these daydreams, I was able-bodied again; I'd never seriously imagined a future in which I was not physically fit and free of pain. Even after getting my power chair, after learning to drive with hand controls, I did not consider myself *disabled* in any permanent sense of the word. I was biding my time, waiting for the day when I'd see the right doctor, find the right medication, make a full recovery.

As a result, I experienced my day-to-day life with a curious sense of distance. It was if I was watching myself, or a person like myself, someone who was holding my place in the world, keeping up appearances until my real self could return. The final semester I spent at the University of Maine, completing the anthropology degree I'd settled on during my medical leave, only reinforced that feeling of disconnection, of being both me and not-me. The people I'd known had all graduated and gone. The places I'd most loved—the Northeast Archives of Folklore and Oral History, the weekly vegetarian cafe, even the dorm where I'd once lived—were all inaccessible to wheelchairs. As soon as the snow started to fall, campus plows buried the curb cuts so I couldn't get to the cafeteria, to classes, to the health center where I was supposed to be working with a physical therapist. The university's solution, instead of plowing the cuts, was to have other students bring me food, books, and missed assignments. Mornings, I looked out my window at a campus that might as well have been a photograph. When I met with the university president to discuss the problems I'd been having, he bluffed and blustered like a football coach, urged me not to give up, reminded me that when the going gets tough, the tough get going. Then—to illustrate his point, I suppose—he hustled me out the door.

Still, by the end of December, I had my degree in hand. In addition to this degree, I had also acquired a boyfriend, a nice and decent boyfriend, who no one in my family trusted, least of all me, because if he really was such a nice and decent boyfriend and not some weirdo with a Florence Nightingale complex, then why was he going out with me? I couldn't walk more than a few steps, I couldn't use my hands very well, and I was in so much pain that I couldn't concentrate from one minute to the next. If I picked up my car keys, I might manage to put them in my purse, but it was just as likely I'd find them, hours later, in the freezer.

Dialing the phone, I'd forget who I was calling and have to ask, Who is this? The pain was worse at night; I lay awake for hours on my flat dorm mattress, pillows wedged between my knees so my legs wouldn't press against each other. Even without a bed frame, the mattress took up a third of the room. During the day, I navigated by pulling myself backward across the floor on my butt, because the space the university had assigned me was too small for the Death Star to maneuver.

This was how I'd greeted my nice and decent boyfriend when he arrived at my door to pick me up for our first date.

At first, I was nervous, but I forgot all about that when I realized I couldn't remember his name. We had tickets to a campus production of *Ain't Misbehavin',* and on the way over to the auditorium, I sneaked glances at his shoes (high-topped tennies), his clothes (what we called *granola,* a cross between hippie and grunge), his face (high cheekbones, wide gray eyes), hoping that something would ring a bell. Distracted, I veered toward a curb cut and accidentally rolled over his foot.

"It didn't hurt," he said. He was limping, but just a little bit.

When we got to the auditorium, we were hustled into "special seating," a row of folding chairs lined up behind the affixed seats. An older man with his foot in a cast was already there. Clearly, he thought my nice and decent boyfriend was a paid assistant. Ignoring me altogether, he fixed my nice and decent boyfriend with an oddly imploring gaze and asked, "Have we met before? What's your name?" Jake's answer solved one problem, but established another: the man would not stop talking. Each time Jake turned back to me, the man would ask him another question, and these questions were becoming increasingly personal when the lights dimmed and the curtain rose and the singing and dancing began.

I'm not sure how much time had passed before I noticed that the man had put his arm around the back of Jake's chair.

I waited for some reaction on Jake's part, but there was none. True, his expression seemed a bit peculiar, as if he were holding his breath, but he didn't move away. Suddenly I felt sad and tired and confused. I'd *thought* this was a date—Jake had been appearing, accidentally on purpose, in the lobby of my dorm for weeks—but now I wasn't sure. For all I knew, hanging out with crippled women was a great way to meet guys, like taking a dog to the park. Besides, I'd suspected his motives all along. He'd just felt sorry for me. Or worse, he was doing this on a dare or a bet. Or even worse still, he wanted to tell me all about the healing love of Our Lord Jesus Christ. In September, after I had eaten alone in the cafeteria for weeks, a girl I recognized from one of my classes had sat down beside me, said hello, and then told me sweetly and brightly that if I came to her church and said, "I accept Jesus Christ as my savior," I could throw away my wheelchair forever.

I started to laugh, I couldn't help it, thinking about what a wheelchair like mine had cost.

"Don't you think," I asked the girl, "we should donate it to the VA instead?"

I saw the man's hand, pale as a dove, take flight in the darkness. Down and down it came until it landed on Jake's thigh.

How grateful I am, now, to that odd, lonely stranger. Without his persistence, I doubt Jake would have touched me. *I* certainly wouldn't have touched him. And if we hadn't touched, we would have been forced to rely on words alone, and words alone would have failed us miserably and completely. We would have made stilted small talk, said good night, gone our separate ways. Instead, in a single fluid motion, Jake scooted his folding chair away from the man and took my hand firmly in his.

It was a warm hand, rough and broad, the palm once and again the size of mine. The weight of it stunned me. An anchor had fallen into my lap, into my life, and I held on for all I was worth.

The man stared at us—at me—with disbelief. Then he hobbled away, faceless angel, into the immortal light of our past.

At intermission, still holding hands, we left the auditorium and wandered across the campus. It was late October, almost Halloween. The night sky was glossy, swollen with a harvest moon, and the sidewalks shouted with leaves. Back at my dorm room, we carved a jack-o'-lantern, and drank from the bottle of Irish whiskey Jake happened to have in his coat pocket, and told each other pretty much everything we'd need to know for the rest of our lives. Just before daybreak, he put on his coat and carried the jack-o'-lantern outside, where he left it, burning, in the icy fork of a tree. From my window, it seemed to be suspended in the air, grinning madly, a rogue miracle. It caught me off guard. It burned through my detachment, stung me with my own loneliness, and longing, and hope.

So now I had this boyfriend. I had parents who would have given their own lives to salvage the spectacular wreckage of mine. And, unbelievably, I had been offered something of a future. Just before graduation, one of my professors took me aside and told me that he needed a graduate assistant to help with a study of plasmids, the DNA that occurs outside the nucleus of the cell. He would, he said, take care of all the paperwork. By January, I'd be a full-time graduate student, with a reasonable stipend and health benefits. In five years, I'd have my Ph.D. in biology. I'd be qualified for a good lab job.

When I told my parents about it, they were beside themselves with joy.

I shouldn't have told my parents about it.

As graduation loomed, I grew more and more uneasy about the assistantship. Clearly, the professor had made an opening in his lab especially for me, and there was such compassion in his eyes whenever he spoke to me that I knew I couldn't bear working for him, couldn't endure such kindness. Besides, *plasmid* was an ugly word. I couldn't say it aloud without feeling I'd stepped in something awful.

At the end of the semester, I refused the assistantship.

I enrolled in a creative writing class at the University of Southern Maine.

Jake already had a job in Portland, working for a small advertising circular. Soon after we moved to the little town of Saco, I began applying for a series of jobs I wouldn't get.

"That position has just been filled," said the woman behind the desk at the hair salon, and she took the RECEPTIONIST WANTED sign out of the window. The next day, driving by, Jake and I saw that it was back. By now, we were not surprised. In the past, I'd worked at a variety of odd jobs—receptionist, salesclerk, waitress, theater usher—but it was clear that I was not going to be hired for even those positions I could physically handle. My anthropology degree had left me unqualified for any salaried profession I could think of. My musical training was useless to me now. Why hadn't I majored in something useful? How was I ever going to support myself?

Our ground-floor apartment had electric heat and sat directly on a concrete slab. Though we kept the thermostat at fifty-eight, our electric bills were nearly twice what we'd budgeted for groceries. As soon as the sun went down, we went to bed and stayed there, reading and talking under a down-filled quilt Jake's mother had given us for Christmas. All night long, trucks screamed past on I-95, headlights slashing the darkness over our heads. Mornings, we blew frost angels at each other over the breakfast table. We had looked at dozens of other apartments, but this had been our only option. It was the only place we'd found with a level entrance for a wheelchair.

Neither of us had health insurance. I didn't have a doctor or a physical therapist. When I finally ran out of anti-inflammatories, I didn't get a new prescription, and I didn't go back to the clinic for cortisone shots. Oddly enough, I found I didn't feel any worse than before. In fact, my stomach felt better, and without the constant irritation of physical therapy, I was able to stand up longer, to shower without holding on to the wall, to crutch between the bedroom and the kitchen instead of relying on the wheelchair. There were times when, sitting quietly, I'd realize I wasn't in quite as much pain. I could hold a full cup of tea, lift it to my mouth again and again; I could balance an open book in my lap, turn a chapter's worth of pages. And, with braces, I could type fairly well, using my thumb and index fingers.

Three times a week, two hours at a time, I bundled up in the Christmas quilt and sat—writing and resting and writing—at the desk Jake had rigged for me out of cinder blocks and an unfinished wood door. There I tried my best to shuck off my body, determined to abandon the present as well as the past, to enter into a whole new world that had absolutely nothing to do with me. I was going to write *fiction.* I was going to get famous, make a lot of money, pay off all my debts. In the process, I would become somebody else altogether, a person I'd invented, successful, sophisticated, interesting.

I decided to hone my writing skills on a short story or two before diving into a full-fledged novel. The trouble was that I couldn't recall ever reading a short story I'd liked, though there'd been plenty that had left me cold, or annoyed, or feeling like the little boy in the tale "The Emperor's New Clothes." Was everybody really seeing all that stuff about symbolism and metaphor, about the universal human condition, or were they just pretending it was there, afraid to admit they disagreed? I disagreed. My English classes had inevitably centered on stories about safaris, or wars, or jolly old England, and though I could accept that such conditions were human, they were not universal, and they were not mine. It seemed to me that my life, like the lives of the people I knew, was something that happened on one planet, and Great Literature was something that happened on another, and that these two planets—though briefly visible to one another every once in a great while—had amazingly little in common. Reading men like Hemingway and F. Scott Fitzgerald made me feel as if some vast, amorphous god were taking an eraser to my life, my individual beliefs and concerns. In the margins of Henry James's *The Golden Bowl,* I'd scrawled, "If these people had to work for a living, it wouldn't matter whether or not the stupid bowl was cracked."

So why, then, were my own first stories clumsy imitations of James, of Fitzgerald, of the very writers I'd most fervently disliked?

I wrote the way I thought I was supposed to write, setting my stories in exotic locations, rendering them in highly Latinate diction. Because who would want to read about people who sounded, well, average? About people who talked like my family, like me? My characters didn't merely roll out of bed, head to the bathroom, and wash their faces in the morning; they *arose and adjourned to the lavatory to perform their morning ablutions.* The men hunted and smoked cigars; the women wore silk and sipped Pernod, which I couldn't pronounce and had never tasted. Everybody had long discussions about the pointlessness, the meaninglessness, of everything. People "just shrugged" a lot and said, "I don't care." Then they committed strange, violent acts. Narrators were particularly inclined to kill themselves when the story was written in the first person.

Needless to say, all of my characters were able-bodied and beautiful.

My creative writing teacher was a gentle person. After reading one of my early stories, she said that, sometimes, she read things which were so painful, so disturbing, that she locked them up in a part of her brain where she knew she'd never encounter them again.

"I don't know what else to write about," I said.

"Write about what you know," she said. "Write about things you *care* about." She told me that Flannery O'Connor once wrote that anybody with a childhood had enough material to write good fiction.

"Who is Flannery O'Connor?" I said.

The night after I first read O'Connor's story "Good Country People," I dreamed that she and I met for lunch in a school cafeteria. In life, she'd struggled with a mysterious ailment that eventually was diagnosed as lupus; it killed her in 1964, the same year I was born. In my dream, she was on crutches, and I was in my power chair. Her hair was flaming orange and teased into a tall beehive. I followed her through the line as she piled food on her tray, speaking irritably to the servers, pointing at what she wanted. Without looking back to see if I was coming, she *picked up her tray and crutched*—gracefully, without dropping the tray or spilling anything—toward an empty table. "How did you do that?" I said, stunned. She made an impatient gesture with her head, as if to say *duh,* then started in on her lunch. My manuscripts were stacked beside her plate, but she didn't seem to notice them, and when she'd finished eating, she stood up to go.

"Aren't you going to tell me what you think about my stories?" I said.

O'Connor waved her hand dismissively at the manuscripts. "Yes, yes, yes," she said. She was already moving away. "It's all very well and good. But *what* are you trying to *say?*"

I woke up. It seemed like a reasonable question. I had no idea how to answer it.

My teacher assigned what she called *springboard exercises* at the end of every class.

Write about a secret.

Write about a pet.

Describe your earliest memory.

These exercises were meant to launch us into stories, but they only served to launch me into full-fledged despair. Night after night, I sat at my desk without writing anything, aside from a fresh row of scratch-outs on the surface of the unfinished door. Whenever my wrists got too sore to type, I jotted notes this way—reminders more than words—in a shorthand I'd invented. I still couldn't hold a pen, so I used a brace meant for quadriplegics. When my right hand wore out, I'd switch hands; I had a second, left-handed brace for that purpose. You could always tell which scratches had been made by which hand, and all of them looked angry. These springboard exercises were stupid. How was I supposed to recall my childhood when I couldn't even come up with details about the past few years, the past few weeks? I forgot deadlines, dates, assignments; sometimes, I'd forget the day of the week. When that happened, I'd panic completely. I'd feel myself falling, as if in a dream: Who am I? How can all of this have come to be? What will happen next?

My legs hurt, my arms hurt, and I'd started to develop what would become chronic back problems from sitting so much of the time. Though I often reminded myself that things were better than they had been, the pain was still distracting, like the wail of an infant in a nearby room. Even after all this time, I could never completely block it out. Even after all this time, I couldn't fully believe that any of this had happened to me, was happening to me, my god, this was my *life* and what was I going to do?

"Can I help?" Jake said from the door. He knew that I was hating my English lit class, which I'd had to take in order to be eligible for my creative writing class. He knew that my creative writing class wasn't going very well at all.

"Not really," I said.

"I wish I could do something," he said, and I could tell how very much he meant it.

That night I wrote a story in which a man admits to his ill and unhappy wife that he is helpless to console her. My teacher liked it better than anything of mine she'd read before.

I wrote another story in which an old man digs a series of holes in his backyard, trying to escape his own increasing sense of disorientation. My teacher pointed out that it dealt with themes of entrapment, frustration, physical restraint. I hadn't meant to write about my own situation, but there it was. My writing was changing. I was changing. Each time I wrote, I found more of myself embedded in the prose: things I remembered that I'd thought I'd forgotten, things I had felt that I hadn't known I was feeling. Each time I went to my desk, I became a little more attached to the world.

Describe your childhood kitchen.

List the contents of your top dresser drawer.

Write a concrete scene that implies an abstract emotion: anger, despair, curiosity, peace.

Winter passed. The weather warmed. One night in late April, writing late with the window cracked to the sound of peepers trilling in the ditches, I stumbled upon the litany

I'd chanted as a child in Michigan, strings of words that swelled and sang, unspooling onto the page. There were the rooms of our rented house, my brother in his crib. There was the Infant of Prague, the picnic table built into the wall. I wrote until I had it all back, my wrists numb, pain grinding up the backs of my elbows. And yet, I had found a way to transcend it. It wasn't a part of the world I was seeing. It wasn't the story I wanted to tell.

At last, I turned off the computer for the night. I took the power chair into the kitchen, where I reached the ice tray down from the freezer, emptied it into the kitchen sink, and turned on the faucet—just as I'd done throughout my adolescence, after a long day at the piano. As the ice cubes hissed and spat, I remembered that time as well: the silence in my head after the music stopped, the humming in my forearms and hands, the darkness beyond the sliding door off the kitchen, overlooking a ravine. On warm nights, my arms still wet, I'd slip out into the moonlight and follow my shadow into the trees, feeling my way down and down into the gully, then rising again toward the field that led toward the stand of willows, the river, the cow pasture on the other side. It was there for me still, all of it was there. And it was me, now, standing in that field on two strong legs, breathing in the good earth smell of the fast-moving water, splinters of moonlight riding the hard current.

Perhaps, there was nothing permanently wrong with my

memory. Perhaps it was just that I'd lost more than I wanted to remember. Perhaps I simply didn't want to face what I now understood was the truth: that I'd probably never have a clear diagnosis. That I'd have to spend the rest of my life this way, in limbo.

When I was a child, the infant brother of a classmate died unexpectedly. The child had been unbaptized, only two days old. In catechism, Sister Justina explained that an unbaptized person, even a good person, even a little baby, could not go to heaven. No, when such a person died, their soul went into the state of Limbo, a place that was no place, nothing, neither punishment nor reward.

I imagined a gray room without walls, a gray floor, a gray bench. The light was such that there could be no shadow. The temperature of the air would be exactly the temperature of your own skin. You wouldn't know how long you'd been in that room, or how you came to be there, or how much longer you had to go.

Eleven

This is the story that for many years, I wasn't supposed to tell, the single thing my father asked me not to write about.

My father was released from the Rocky Knoll Tuberculosis Sanitarium in October 1956. He was twenty-one years old. Half of one lung had been surgically removed, and the scar—a fine red line that ran beneath his left shoulder blade—itched relentlessly. He'd become something of a favorite on the ward, and on the morning he was discharged, people lined up to say their good-byes. My grandfather, who'd arrived alone, waited downstairs in the lobby, shifting his feet in their mud-caked boots. He'd already been out to the fields that morning and was anxious to get back home. Already the new season's work was beginning. Already there was more to be done than a man could do in a day, particularly a man with one son gone into the navy and the other out of shape, winded by the walk to the car.

What did they talk about on the way home, my grandmother's absence sleeping between them like a difficult child nobody wants to wake? What did my father feel as they passed back into Ozaukee county, turned onto roads that he recognized? Dirty gray crumbles of snow filled the ditches and blurred the edges of the fields. In another few weeks, if the weather held, the earth would be dry enough to cultivate, and then would come the planting, the fertilizing and irrigating, another wave of planting so the harvests could be staggered into late summer and fall. My father had lived all his life by these rhythms, as deeply ingrained as the rhythms of his body, yet it seemed to him now that he'd fallen out of step in a way that could never be reconciled. He knew just as well as his father knew that he was no good for the fields anymore. How was he going to make a living? What was he going to do?

When they got home, my grandfather dropped him off at the house before continuing on down the lane that led toward the woods. My father looked up at the house and barn, which he and his brother had always kept painted. He looked at the clover field sloping down from the house to the highway, a field that, at eighteen, he'd tiled for drainage by hand over the course of a long and grueling summer. He looked at the long, low tool shed he'd built. Perhaps it had been someone else who'd done these things. Perhaps the things he thought he remembered were, in fact, just wistful imaginings. My grandfather's car had already disappeared, dust rising behind it in a lazy strip. A couple of hawks circled high overhead. In the distance, the lake was so clear and blue that it was hard to tell where the horizon ended, where the sky began.

Inside the house, my father sat down at the kitchen table. My grandmother had gone out—for the day, my grandfather had said. Everything looked the same. There was a newspaper and my father picked it up but then he put it down again. For a while, he scratched at his scar; there was no one to tell him to stop. Then he got up and dragged his bag up the stairs to his bedroom. It, too, was exactly as it had been. As if no one had entered it since that January day when he'd packed his things, not knowing if and when he would ever return to this house.

But why wasn't my grandmother there to meet him? Why hadn't she come to visit him in the san?

"Well," my father says. He is standing in my doorway, halfway in and halfway out. He jams his hands deep in his pockets and rattles all his loose change. His body, backlit by the hallway light, is a dark, featureless shape, and the answers he gives to my questions are very much the same. Long before I begin to write fiction, I will learn to fill in these shapes as best I can. I'll burn the facts, the dry, seasoned kindling, and explore whatever truths I can find by their light. I'll add missing colors, textures, and emotions, trying my best to stay within the lines.

Three years into a future I cannot imagine, my father will ask me not to write about his time in the san. It is not that any of this is a secret. It is simply the sort of thing that people, nice people, don't discuss. My father is a respected businessman, and here in our small community, illness and shame go hand in hand. Shame because, if you'd only tried harder, you might have fought off whatever it was that ailed you. Shame because, if you'd lived your life right, God would have protected you, would have answered your prayers, would have kept you safe to begin with. There must have been a moment—one you could have controlled or prevented—when you let down your guard, looked the wrong way, indulged in some slight weakness that opened the door to what was to come.

Even now, far from home, I am able to understand. Haven't I heard these same overtones in the advice of holistic practitioners, in the comments of New Age acquaintances, who suggest that I'm blocking my own healing energy, that maybe I simply don't want to get well? Aren't I regularly approached by Christians who want to know if

I've prayed to Jesus, if I've asked him to forgive my sins? Once, at a party, I noticed a woman staring at me hard, her arms crossed over her chest. "Man, you must have done something *awful* in your last life," she told me, "to deserve what you're going through."

Oh, yes, I understand.

"A writer's only responsibility is to his art," Faulkner wrote. "He will be completely ruthless if he is a good one. He has a dream. It anguishes him so much he must get rid of it. He has no peace until then. Everything goes by the board: home, pride, decency, security, happiness, all to get the book written. If a writer has to rob his own mother, he won't hesitate; the 'Ode to a Grecian Urn' is worth any number of old ladies."

If your soul is flat as the paper you write on, it will cost nothing to agree. But put an honored face on Faulkner's "old lady" and suddenly things aren't so clear. Every writer struggles to find a balance between the paralysis that results from trying to please everyone and the impact of art upon the very lives that inspire it. And while some writers, like Faulkner, do write from a place of loneliness, drunkenness, pain—the stereotype of the angst-stricken artist—there are plenty of us who write best, as I do, from a place of relative well-being. The truth is that I don't write well when I'm unhappy or anxious. I don't write well when my conscience is bothering me. Before my illness, my father was, in many ways, a stranger, and the stories he told me about his illness formed the first bridge between us. And so I chose to endure Faulkner's anguish, rather than get rid of it. For eleven years, I kept the promise I made to my father.

At first, this promise was an easy one to keep. For one thing, nobody wanted to publish the stories I was writing, and I had no reason to believe that this situation would ever change. I told myself that even if I *did* write about my father's experiences, no one would be the wiser for it. For another thing, I had already begun to notice that the more my writing improved, the less satisfied I was with anything I wrote. Soon, fearing acceptance more than rejection, I stopped submitting work for publication, and it was then that I began to write the way I'd once played the piano, the way I once had prayed—with an unabashed, single-minded passion that I found hard to explain. I wrote for myself, out of wonder and fascination, in the absolute freedom of anonymity. And in doing do, I rediscovered the spirituality I thought had been lost along with my Catholicism. Only now, that spirituality was articulated in a new way. Where, once, I would have altered my perceptions of the world to fit the contours of my faith, I now shaped narrative worlds that reflected my honest perceptions—worlds filled with contradictions and blurred edges. Worlds defined by questions rather than answers. Worlds that often served as windows into a larger sense of mystery.

Absolute attention is prayer. Simone Weil's definition is still the most generous I've heard. And when I write, I pay attention. When I write, I focus, I give everything I have. When I write, I move beyond my body, the crippled here and now, to enter a place of greater perspective, where fragmented things become whole—the same transcendence I'd sought through conventional faith. I do not mean to suggest that since such faith didn't happen to lead me there, it is not a road worth taking. But there are as many ways to experience transcendence as there are people in the world, and what brings out the best in one person may leave another person smug, or mean-spirited, or afraid. Perhaps, when we speak of *the meaning of life,* we are talking about our search to find whatever it might be that unlocks our particular heart. And it might be outright worship, but it might just as easily be the act of raising a child. It might be making a quilt, or restoring an antique car, or planting a garden. It might be as simple as the preparation of a meal. I myself am most capable of transcendence when I claim responsibility not only for my failures and limitations but for my triumphs, for my best intentions, for the things that I've done right. And writing allows me to do just that. My characters are the worst and the best of me; there is not one, no matter how mean or glorious, in whom there is nothing I can claim.

Writing has also become the means by which I make

sense of a day-to-day world that doesn't. In life, I'm the sort of person who always comes up with the perfect thing I should have said several hours *after* a conversation has taken place, usually during the middle of the night as I play the scene back, revising it until everything makes sense in a way it never could in life. In life, I forget important names and anniversaries, the location of restaurants, the titles of books I've just read. In life, I am the sort of person who needs to have jokes explained, who hears that a duck has walked into a bar and embraces that image, satisfied. Writing is a way of creating the punch line I have missed, inventing the name I can't remember. Writing is both the necessary map and the X on that map that tells me where I am. When I write, I am able to give myself the last, resonant word. If a duck walks into a bar, that bar belongs to me.

Perhaps this is why the stories I write are inevitably more believable than their factual roots. "Is this about your family?" people ask. Or: "Is that supposed to be me?" It has taken me years to realize that it isn't my scant use of facts that people are reacting to. It's the way I've claimed the last, definitive word on those facts. It's the way those facts have been coaxed into the sort of satisfying shape we long for in our lives, complete with clear motivations, logical developments, resonant closures. It's the way those facts have been illuminated with meaning.

Facts in themselves are as limiting as fences. Why carve up the imagination with all those long, straight lines? I can follow a fence for a while if I must, but inevitably, I hop it, drawn along paths suggested by the contours of the landscape itself. For a while, things resemble my own life, the so-called real world—but then a double moon rises in the sky. By its otherworldly light, I see someone who resembles a dear friend, an imagined lover, a neighbor's child. Five drafts later, fifty drafts later, I understand that I am mistaken. This character is a stranger. This character is astonishing. I have never known, never thought to imagine, anyone like this character before. It is this that keeps me writing, leaves me amazed and humbled again and again. There is always that point—what Flannery O'Connor calls "a moment of grace"—when the sum of the parts becomes larger than the whole.

In 1989, I got a fellowship to attend Cornell University's graduate writing program. Jake and I moved to Ithaca, New York, where, the following year, we were married. By then, I was able to walk unaided around our narrow kitchen; I could comfortably crutch the length of our house. I still needed the power chair to get from the back porch out to the garden, but I weeded the bean rows on my knees and—more important—got back up into the chair afterward. Better still, I was able to hold a regular pen, though my writing was still barely legible, and slow. I had far less pain. I began to gain weight. A teacher introduced me to horseback riding, and I'll alway remember my first time leaving the power chair's rattle to enter the silent, wooded paths beyond the barnyard.

By the end of my second year of graduate school, I'd managed to finish my thesis—a story collection that would eventually become my second published book. In addition, I'd nearly completed what would be my first, something I could no longer pretend was not a novel. *Vinegar Hill* had started out as just another short story, an attempt to reconcile contradictions suggested by details—what Chekhov called "little particulars"—dislodged from the lives of my paternal grandparents. My grandma Ansay had suffered a final, fatal stroke early in 1985. My grandfather now lived in Florida, where he'd gone through a kind of renaissance: dating, taking ballroom dancing classes, blossoming in the sunshine. But I couldn't stop reflecting on the way they had lived: my grandmother's misery, my grandfather's exhaustion, his endless desire for what he called "peace." It occurred to me that like so many farmers of his generation, my grandfather had spent his youth not as a person, but as a tool, a task, the number of hours he could work in a day. His rage, which had simmered far more than it had shown, now seemed to mirror my grandmother's grief—two languages that seemed to express the flip side of a single, shared lament. Perhaps it was this that had kept them together. Perhaps this had something to do with the secret my grandfather knew about my grandmother.

"I'll tell them about you," he'd say, whenever she raised her voice against him.

I never learned what the secret was, but there were several clues. When I was fourteen, my grandmother had pulled me into the bathroom by my wrist. There, speaking through tears, she told me that sex was for the sole purpose of bearing children, and that once I passed out of child-bearing age, I was free to deny a husband anything more. My grandfather had persisted, but she'd known her rights. She'd gone to the priest—on her mother's advice—and the priest had made my grandfather leave her alone.

And then there was this: she'd been past twenty-five, an old maid by the standards of the day, when she'd married. Her father had approached my grandfather, and the two had negotiated until my grandmother's dowry was sweetened with the promise of good land. My grandfather himself had told me the story, in Florida, well after my grandmother's death.

"No one else would have her," he said.

"Why?"

But my grandfather just shook his head. How he loved the Florida sunshine! He went out and bought himself a pale pink suit. He died a happy man.

Vinegar Hill quickly departed from the fragmented facts of my grandparents' lives, entering into the Gothic terrain I'd admired in books by O'Connor and the Brontës. Soon I was enmeshed in a fictional world every bit as real to me as any I had known. I finished the book when I was twenty-five, but I was twenty-eight by the time I'd found a publisher for it, and I'd just turned thirty, and was completing my third book, by the time I finally held the first copy in my hand. It had become the story of woman struggling to reconcile the demands of her faith with the reality of a failing marriage, and, frankly, I lost a lot of sleep, wondering what my Catholic relatives would think of it. In fact, my relatives were overwhelmingly supportive. (I once overheard my Auntie Lu explaining to a stranger at a reading, "When we talk about Ann, we just say, 'the Lord moves in mysterious ways.'") What I had not anticipated—had never even considered—were the reactions I might get from people I didn't know well, people who happened to live in my hometown.

Port Washington, Wisconsin, is a scenic little town of about nine thousand set on a hill overlooking Lake Michigan. People still say "hello" when they pass on the street. At the top of the hill is Saint Mary's Church, an old Catholic church made of stone. Lodged in its steeple is a four-faced clock, one of the largest in the United States. Growing up, it seemed to me that no matter where I was, or who I was with, or what we happened to be doing, the eye of that clock was fixed upon me, unblinking as the eye of God. Who could have resisted such a landscape, so ripe for metaphor? I borrowed the hill, the church, the clock for the fictional town where *Vinegar Hill* is set. I also borrowed my grandparents' house, which resembled many houses in Port Washington, furnished with the same hanging Jell-O molds, the same framed biblical portraits, the same avocado carpeting. I borrowed Lake Michigan—it is, after all, a big lake—and I borrowed a few other general details. A downtown swimming pool, for instance. A tourist-trap restaurant.

Not exactly the town's crown jewels.

I was fully expecting questions about the church and its clock. But what I wasn't expecting was all the people who would accuse me of setting *Vinegar Hill* in *their* home. Who claimed to recognize my protagonist, Ellen, as their own mother, their own best friend, even their own self. Who showed up at the readings I gave in the Milwaukee area to chant the refrain of my childhood: if you can't say something nice, don't say anything at all. In a bookstore, during a question-and-answer exchange, the mother of a childhood friend stood up.

"Nothing like this really happened to you!" she said.

"You're absolutely right," I agreed.

We stared at each other helplessly.

Rumors abounded. A cousin of mine was shown the "real" house where *Vinegar Hill* had taken place—a house I'd never even seen. My parents, who have been married thirty-eight years to date, were whispered to have been *secretly divorced.* My favorite bit of gossip asserted that *Vinegar Hill* was actually "Sweet Cake Hill," a small street in Port Washington I hadn't known existed.

The truth was that I'd struggled to find a title. I'd known early on that it would be the name of the street my characters lived on; I'd known, too, that its connotations should reflect the book's bitter sensibility. And yet, two months after the manuscript was finished, the title page was blank. I was still living in upstate New York, teaching at Cornell as a visiting lecturer. One day, driving out of town to see a friend, I glanced up and saw a street sign I'd never noticed before.

Vinegar Hill.

I leaned on my horn. I zigged and zagged through the autumn leaves. Never since has a title hit me with such absolute clarity.

I once heard another writer say that we are living in a time of such cynicism that all nonfiction is assumed to be fiction and all fiction is assumed to be nonfiction. The fact is that certain people will see themselves in your work, regardless of whether or not you put them there. There will always be the postpublication smirks, the howls of betrayal, the accusations of thievery. In a sense, it's liberating. You're damned if you do, damned if you don't.

And yet, in this case, I'm glad that I didn't.

Halfway through the first draft of *Vinegar Hill*, as I was struggling with a character named James, an entire backstory appeared to me—not exactly based on my father's experience in the san, but springing from it. For nearly a year, I wrote this backstory in, then wrote it back out. Ultimately, I let it go, and to this day, I am grateful. No matter how different James was from my father, no matter how distinct his circumstances might become, the word *tuberculosis* would have had to remain, like a tombstone, like a monument, visible for miles. The effect on my relationship with my father, with my family, would have been devastating. And the effect on my writing? One could argue that I'd be a better writer for the experience. One could also argue that I would not have gone on to write as prolifically, as freely, and with the sense of joy that sustains me, had there been that weight on my conscience, that distracting sting.

As it was, my parents took all the attention, good as well as bad, in stride. My father, a consummate salesman, actually *liked* the controversy over our personal lives, believing that it could only boost sales. At local book signings, I'd see him grinning mischievously when people asked him if the book was about our family.

"Have you read it?" he'd ask.

If the answer was no: "Well, then, you'll have to read it and let me know."

And if they *had* read it?

"Oh, she's got another book coming soon. Once you read that one, it'll clear things up."

My mother was more cryptic. There's a scene in the book where Ellen is playing tumbling games with the children; at one point, she stands on her head. Signing books at a local library fund-raiser, I heard a woman asking my mother, in a stage whisper, if Ellen was supposed to be her.

"Well," my mother said, evenly, "I really can stand on my head."

Between 1994 and 1999, I published four novels and a collection of short stories, statistics that mean I've spent roughly a year of my life on a book tour. Since handicap access to public transportation can be, as my father would say, "a challenge," he arranges to meet me whenever I give readings in the Midwest. He picks me up at O'Hare and chauffeurs me to talks and interviews in the Chicago area before driving me north to Milwaukee, Madison, Minneapolis. We take the backroads, the rural highways he still remembers from when he was just starting out, fresh from the san, working as a traveling salesman selling fertilizer across the Midwest. We listen to polka tapes and AM radio. My father points out how the little towns have changed, admiring the Wal-Marts, the shopping malls, the super-size grocery stores.

"When I used to come through here, there was nothing but cows!" he declares, biting happily into a deli sandwich.

It's early in the evening, July 1996. I've just finished speaking to a book club in Madison, and my father and I are driving north toward Minneapolis, passing between the endless darkening fields. He has been evaluating my response to the book club's questions, pointing out places where my answers were too long, recalling missed opportunities, drawing my attention to a moment when, caught off guard, I made a self-deprecating remark. This postgame analysis might sound unpleasant; it's not. My father's observations are practical ones. He evaluates me the way he might evaluate another experienced salesperson. He evaluates me the way he might evaluate himself.

"The product is good," he says, thumping my latest novel with affection. "If a product is good, it will always sell."

And now we've settled into comfortable silence, polka music chortling from the radio, the last of the sunset lapping the curve of the horizon, when he says, "Are your legs bothering you?"

So they are. I realize I'm wearing what my husband calls my "gray look," the angry, impatient expression I get when I'm in pain. *In pain*—such a maudlin phrase, and yet I'm intrigued by its implications. *In pain,* like a faraway place or a state of mind; like a country where you've gone to live for a while. *In the Arctic Circle. In a state of grace.* My arms are aching, too, particularly my right elbow and wrist. I am right-handed, and everywhere we go, there are books to personalize, stock to sign.

"Tomorrow is a light day for me," I remind us both. I'm scheduled to fly to Seattle in the morning; my next reading isn't till the following night, and I have nothing to do in between except speak to a university class, which is something I particularly enjoy doing. I'm thinking ahead to that, and to San Francisco, where I'll be heading after Seattle, and the friends I hope to see while I'm there, when my father says suddenly, almost savagely, "It's such a shame this had to happen to you."

For a moment, I think he's talking about my writing career, my books. Then I understand. I look at him, at his unrelenting profile, so much like my own. Yes, it is a shame—and no, it is not. It is simply what it is. Meaning is the color of whatever lens we happen to wear when we look at our lives. Like fiction, meaning evolves out of our own fascination and need, a structure we invent from facts that, on their own, would add up to very little. Like fiction, it tells a story that may or may not have anything to do with our lives. Yet if we tell the story well enough, it becomes believable. It becomes true.

"Such a shame," my father says again, and his voice,

which is gentler now, breaks. And I realize he has carried this thought since I first fell ill, a weight every bit as constant, as distracting, as my own physical discomfort. I see him at nineteen, working in his father's fields, so tired that by noon he must return to the house. I watch as he sits down on the porch steps, too weak to go inside. Thinking, What the hell is the matter with me? Thinking, Am I losing my mind?

He entered the san as a young man with prospects; he left at twenty-one, missing most of one lung, with no idea what he would do next. Men his age were heading for Korea. Women his age awaited their return, rings shining on their fingers. He had toppled out of his life the way, someday, I would topple out of mine. He would start over, work his way up from entry-level sales, start his own company. He would fall in love and have children. He would stand in the doorway of his oldest, the excitable one, the one so full of energy that as a child, she'd prowled the house in her sleep, and he'd tell her that someday, she'd look back on this time of stillness and it would be nothing at all. You'll start over, he assured me. You'll catch up. You'll find a way to turn all of this to your advantage.

I remember how he took my photograph—over my protests—sitting in my power wheelchair. "To look back on," he said. "After you get better. After you don't need things like this anymore."

We are hurtling through the absolute country darkness of western Wisconsin: no light pollution, no other cars. There's only the sunburst of our own headlights, illuminating the road just ahead of us, just in time. E. M. Forster said that writing a novel is like driving a car at night with the headlights on: you can't see your final destination, but you can see enough to make the whole trip that way. The truth is this: I do not know my destination. All I know is the circle of light just ahead, its shifting geography. And suddenly, more than anything else in the world, I want to write down what I see. Because it isn't a shame so much as a wonder, if only because it's so far away from anything I might have imagined or dreamed. The way my father's life is different from what he had imagined, coming in from the field, coming home from the san, and thinking it was all over for him when, in fact, it was only beginning.

It is not that I believe the things that happen to us happen for a reason. I certainly don't believe that *things have a way of working out for the best,* something I've been told countless times by well-meaning doctors, family members, and friends. But I do believe that each of us has the ability to decide how we'll react to the random circumstances of our lives, and that our reactions can shape future circumstances, affect opportunities, open doors. The truth is that I love my life, and to love it fully, I must acknowledge that it could not be what it is had I *not* fallen ill. I told my father all of this as we drove toward Minneapolis. I told him how I thought the parallel between our lives was an interesting one, something that I really wanted to write about—in fiction or nonfiction, I wasn't sure. I told him I didn't think I could write about my own experience without including, in some way, his, and the stories he had told me, and what they'd meant to me.

It was the perfect opportunity for him to say he understood, to tell me I was free to write whatever I wanted, with his blessing. If this had been a fictional scene, he would have done so. But in fact, it would be 1998 before he'd call me up, out of the blue, to give me this unexpected gift.

To say that if I wanted to write about his time in the san, I could do so.

Sixteen years have passed since I gave up the piano, since one door shut and a window opened, since I entered the life I am living today. It's a good life, made up of the people I love, the novels I've written and those I plan to write, the students I've taught who have come and gone, the places in the world I have seen and the places I long to go. In four more years, at forty, I will have been disabled for half my life, but although "probable multiple sclerosis" continues to appear on my medical charts, I still do not have a definitive diagnosis. Recently, I've started treatment at an integrative medical center; my physician there believes I'm struggling with an autoimmune disorder brought on by childhood inoculations. Who can say? I have altered my diet, as instructed. I have acupuncture treatments twice a week. I've weaned myself off my latest anti-inflammatory prescription; instead, I swallow fistfuls of nutritional supplements and Chinese herbs.

Is it helping? friends and family want to know.

I tell them that I think so. I tell them that I have to wait and see.

There was a time in my life when I would have said this kind of uncertainty was unbearable. When I believed I could not live without a prognosis, a reliable map by which I might plan out my future. When I believed that an explanation was nothing less than my due. When I fully expected a closure as final, as satisfying, as the end of a Beethoven symphony.

I was formed by a place where the roads met at right angles, a landscape in which cause and effect were visible for miles. I was raised to believe that every question had its single, uniform answer, and that answer was God's will. But the human body, like the life it leads, is ultimately a mystery, and to live my life without restraint, to keep moving forward instead of looking back, I have had to let go of that need to understand *why* what has happened has happened and, indeed, is happening still. In some ways, my health has gotten worse in recent years. My vision blurs when my eyes get tired, and this means I have had to learn a whole new way of writing, arranging ideas in my head, doing the bulk of my work off the page. I've given up movies and watching TV; I read very little; I no longer drive.

On the other hand, the inflammation in my arms and legs has stabilized since my early twenties. As a result, I'm in far less pain. I can write with a pen if I take frequent breaks. I use a scooter instead of a wheelchair, and months will pass in which I'm able to use it for distances only. I can stroll into a restaurant if somebody pulls the car up to the door. I can pace a few laps in a swimming pool, provided I don't do it every day. But I've learned not to take such luxuries for granted. Without warning, I can have flareups, bad spells that can last weeks, even months. During those times, night pain keeps me from sleeping, and I move through the day as if in a cloud, relying on the scooter for everything I do. Motion and light leave my head aching; I write in ten-minute snatches, the font size set at sixteen. These are the times I need stiff wrist supports to type, to handle silverware, to hold a telephone receiver to my ear. These are the times I wake up in the morning and wrap my ankles and elbows and knees before hauling myself out of bed. These are the times when it's hard not to dwell on the larger issue at hand: what if I don't snap out of it this time? What is going to happen next?

Yet, in one way or another, this is everybody's question,

and one of life's few consistent blessings is that we cannot know the future. At any moment, all that we claim as our own might be instantly swept away. But perhaps it's this precarious balance that drives us to value what we have, to cling to the world as we do. And isn't it all we do not know that constitutes possibility?

I think of the ancient mapmakers charting the flat reaches of the world. *Here there be dragons,* they wrote along the edges of the known continents, warning ships away from the uncharted waters beyond. No doubt there could be dragons, and worse, out in the mist. But one might just as easily sketch an island of flowers, rainbows, and flying fish, wonders that have yet to be imagined.

This, then, is the map of my own making. This is the story I am learning to live.